MARATHONING *for* MORTALS

A REGULAR PERSON'S GUIDE TO THE JOY OF RUNNING OR WALKING A HALF-MARATHON OR MARATHON

JOHN "THE PENGUIN" BINGHAM,
RUNNER'S WORLD columnist and author of *No Need for Speed,*
and
Coach JENNY HADFIELD, M.A., C.P.T.

RODALE

© 2003 by John Bingham and Jenny Hadfield

All rights reserved. No part of this publication may be reproduced or transmitted in any form or by any means, electronic or mechanical, including photocopying, recording, or any other information storage and retrieval system, without the written permission of the publisher.

Runner's World is a registered trademark of Rodale Inc.

Printed in the United States of America
Rodale Inc. makes every effort to use acid-free ∞, recycled paper ♻.

Interior design by Christina Gaugler

Library of Congress Cataloging-in-Publication Data

Bingham, John, date.
    Marathoning for mortals : a regular person's guide to the joy of
running or walking a half-marathon or marathon / John "The Penguin"
Bingham and Jenny Hadfield.
        p.   cm.
    Includes index.
    ISBN 1–57954–782–6 paperback
    1. Marathon running—Training.   I. Hadfield, Jenny.   II. Title.
GV1065.17.T73B53   2003
796.42'52—dc21   2003000217

Distributed to the book trade by St. Martin's Press

6   8   10   9   7   5   paperback

Visit us on the Web at www.runnersworld.com, or call us toll-free at (800) 848-4735.

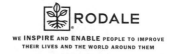

To the patient heroes of Team in Training, for teaching us to accept life's challenges with grace and courage.

Contents

Part Four: Game Face

Training Plans

Acknowledgments

We don't know where most books are written, but we suspect that more often than not the messiness of the creative process takes place in private. Our lives would not allow for that, and so nearly every word of this book was written in full public view.

With that in mind, we'd like to thank the management and staff of the Hampton Inn in Bellingham, Washington. They understood the paradox of two people sitting on the sofa all day and eating while writing a book about the benefits of an active, healthy lifestyle.

We'd like to thank, too, our friends and neighbors at the Melrose Restaurant in Chicago's Lakeview area. They tolerated us occupying a table for hours at a time while we jammed on our laptops. Their food fed our bodies, and their kindness and encouragement nourished our spirits.

Specifically, we'd like to thank Mike Norman of Chicago Endurance Sports for his help with the Cross-Training chapter, Alex McKinney of Athletico for his help with the Injury Prevention chapter, and Dave Zimmer, Lisa Zimmer, and Sabra Bederka of Fleet Feet Chicago and Julie Leasure of Nike for their help with the Gear chapter. Their contributions were invaluable in providing technical expertise, solid advice, and common sense.

Jenny in particular thanks her mother and father for supporting her never-ending attempts to reach for the stars; Wendy for being a great sister; her brothers, Scott and Don, for being her biggest fans; and the "third-floor gang" for feeding her when she was hungry and listening to the ups and downs in her life.

She also thanks Kathy O'Malley for being an incredible role model and Yvette Arnoux for being a great listener and spiritual guide.

—⚹⚹—

Beyond the usual suspects, like the incomparable folks at *Runner's World* US and UK, there have been a number of gray eminences who quietly contributed to our ability to start this project and have been staunch supporters as we've worked our way through to its completion. They are too modest to want to be named but they know who they are—and so do we.

No list of thank-you's would be complete without acknowledging Alisa Bauman. She is a skilled editor and gifted collaborator. The significance of her contribution cannot be overstated.

Most important, we'd like to thank the thousands of walkers and runners that we've encountered in our personal and professional lives. We want to thank each and every one of them for their honesty and openness, for their willingness to include us in their successes, and for all the laughter and tears that we have shared at the finish lines. Our lives have been enhanced by their strength, determination, and joy.

Last but not least, thanks to the cutest dog in the world, Bear, for riding endless miles in the backpack and spending countless hours alone in the apartment, yet always managing to greet us with tail-wagging enthusiasm!

Foreword

During what I would term the first wave of the "running boom" in the 1970s and '80s, the concern of many runners, if not most, was to set personal records—to train harder and harder, race faster and faster. Experts and amateurs treated the sport like an elite club that wouldn't have them unless they shaved seconds daily. In 2003, many of those people are still running with the same mind-set. If they have managed to hold together orthopedically, God bless them.

But for most of us, running isn't that way anymore. We are part of a new wave that began in the mid-1990s. We are more moderate. Some of us are even involved in training a new generation, running for what I term "other people and other reasons." Everyone is welcome now. Personally, I am happy to see the club disbanded.

This second wave has leaders, too, but their goals are far more realistic and attainable. Take the authors of this book: Two decades ago, who would have taken instruction from a penguin or a gym-class dropout?

Today, though, John "the Penguin" Bingham and Jenny Hadfield are bringing marathons to the masses. They remind us that a big part of running—the part where the fun and personal gratification are kept—is the journey. They know that simply finishing a marathon can be one of life's personal joys.

So if joy is what you want, we've found your coaches. Allow John and Jenny to demystify running. Let them show you how the mortals marathon. You may never win in New York or Boston, but the race for fulfillment will be yours hands down. And that may be the sweetest victory known.

—**Frank Shorter,** *1972 Olympic-marathon gold medalist and 1976 Olympic-marathon silver medalist*

Introduction

You already have everything you need to be a long-distance athlete. It's mind-set—not miles—that separates those who do from those who dream.

—〜〜—

There's a story about a hungry man who walks into the market square with only a pot full of water and a pocket full of stones. As he sets his pot on the fire to boil the water, a curious crowd gathers.

"What are you making?" ask the onlookers.

"Stone soup," he replies. "I really like stone soup," he continues, "but some carrots would sure make it better."

Someone produces carrots. "And celery, too; that makes it better." Soon, he has celery as well. The story goes on, and the man ends up with a soup complete with vegetables and meat.

Starting a long-distance training program is a lot like making stone soup. Right now, it may not seem like you have very much. You may not be in the best shape of your life (and therefore, your fitness has been "watered down"). You may weigh more than you wish (your pot). You may even think that your personal genetics ill suit you for long-distance running or walking (your stones). Well, you've come to the right place.

We haven't found a mortal who couldn't run a half- or full marathon. You already have everything you need to be a long-distance athlete. You see, once you decide to run or walk farther than the 10-K (6.2 miles), your quest centers much more on tenacity than talent. Even the very best athletes at the 20-K, half-

1

marathon, or full-marathon distance will tell you that the mind-set—not the miles—separates those who finish long-distance events from those who only dream of finishing.

So bring the pot, the water, and the stones. We'll supply the carrots, celery, assorted other vegetables, and meat. We'll help you turn your stone soup into a stellar supper.

A Program for Every Mortal

Training books, even the best of them, tend to try to find the least common denominator among runners and walkers and then describe formulas that work for as many folks as possible. What we've found, in observing and coaching thousands of people, is that there is no least common denominator. Each of us comes with a unique history, a unique biology, and a unique set of skills and experiences.

That's why you won't find any formulas in *Marathoning for Mortals*. This is not a rulebook. It won't tell you everything you have to do and all the things you mustn't do.

Instead, you'll find training tools, training plans, lots of helpful hints, and the wisdom of dozens of long-distance athletes who have personally conquered the half- and full-marathon distances. You'll find eight different training programs, including pure running plans, run/walk plans, and simple walking plans for the half- and full-marathon distances. But you won't find any formulas. You'll find only strategies that will help you discover your own course to the finish line.

We wrote our training programs with the help of the running and walking community. Rather than try to create a plan that works well for a few and not at all for most, we've chosen to give you all the information you need to design a plan that works for you, for your level of interest and experience, in your life as you have to live it.

So you've never run a step before in your life? No problem. One of our plans will work for you. You've already completed a marathon but want to run your next one a little bit faster? We've got a program that will work for you, too.

You really want to complete a marathon, but you're worried that your knee pain will act up? We've got a program for that. You feel silly every time you run but you've always dreamed of going the distance? We've got something that will work.

It doesn't matter where you're coming from. It doesn't matter how un-divine your running skills are. It doesn't matter how low you feel you rank among the ranks of mortals. You can and will become a long-distance athlete. We promise. We've seen it happen. We've seen mortals of every shape and size, of every type of fitness background, of every sort of lifestyle cross the marathon finish line.

You can be one of them. We invite you to experience the joy that many of us find as the miles we run exceed the miles we thought we could run.

In Part One, you'll learn everything you need to know about yourself to get started. Many new long-distance athletes skip this important first step in their long-distance training programs and suffer disastrous results as a consequence. Your past injuries, your current health and fitness status, your lifestyle, and your personality will all help to determine the best training plan and race goal for you.

In Part Two, you'll discover the method behind the training madness. Each chapter will teach you about the key workouts and their sequence and intensity level. These chapters will provide the blueprint that you need to successfully follow the right training program for you and to alter that program to fit your personal needs.

In Part Three, you'll find important tools to help keep your training on track. Injury prevention, cross-training, nutrition, and gear all help to keep you comfortable, pain-free, energetic, and motivated to continue to forge ahead.

In Part Four, you'll learn everything you need to know about the race itself. You'll find out how to motivate yourself from the start to the finish—and beyond. From dealing with prerace jitters to postfinish letdown, we'll take you on a step-by-step journey that will prepare you for every step to marathon success.

Last but not least, at the end of the book, you'll find eight different training plans, ranging in distance and difficulty from walking a half-marathon to running a full marathon. You'll follow the training program most suited to your background, personality, and goals.

We recommend that you read the entire book before taking your first step. Then during your training, keep the book nearby. You will encounter obstacles. You will ask questions. You can return to the book again and again to help you sort out the causes and cures for aches and pains and motivation lapses.

This book marks the sum of years of race expo lectures, training clinics, training programs, and workouts. It is a compilation of seasoned half- and full marathoners' tips, race directors' advice on how to tackle a long-distance course, and the questions that we have heard over and over through the years.

We hope that it serves to guide you physically, mentally, and spiritually through a life full of race stories and dreams realized. Once you realize those dreams, we hope you pass this book on to a friend who shares the same fears, a friend who is looking for that same glimmer of hope.

Who We Are

We're runners and writers who have conquered the mystery of the distance, over and over and over again. We've also stood as witnesses to thousands of others who have also triumphed over their own fears. We've coached runners from their first steps all the way to the finish line.

John's Background

Most people know me by my nickname, "the Penguin." I earned that nickname by starting my active life at 240 pounds (about 90 more than I weigh now). As I ran one day, I caught a glimpse of myself in a storefront window. Unlike the thin, agile runner that I had envisioned I was, I instead saw a short, fat man waddling down the sidewalk. In one instant, the Penguin was born.

Since those early days of struggling with an overambitious spirit and an underambitious body, I've learned that moving that body with my own two feet has given me more joy, more frustration, and ultimately more knowledge than anything else I'd ever done. Even the years I spent as a professional musician and college professor never gave me the satisfaction that I found in running and walking.

As best as I can figure, I'd be back selling used cars by now if I hadn't met Jenny at a running camp. Oddly enough, I attended that camp as a clinician and she as a participant. In time, though, it was clear that the student was the teacher.

Jenny's Background

I was not a natural-born runner. I always felt embarrassed during gym class because I was the slowest kid in the class. I hated running.

Instead, I participated in team sports. I started 16-inch softball when the ball was bigger than my head. Volleyball and basketball were part of my daily agenda. I ran as a form of punishment. I made myself run five laps if I missed a serve or ten laps for a missed free throw. I quickly associated running laps as a negative outcome in life, a payment for failure.

I dreamed of running normally, running as fast as the other kids and without pain or embarrassment. Every once in a while I would *try* to run normally. I'd strap on my new Nike (Forrest Gump) shoes, set out on the sidewalk, and go. I'd get to the end of the long block and then hang my head and cry all the way home.

I continued to dream of running normally right through college and, as a result, earned a few degrees in exercise physiology. I wanted to teach and coach people how to be active, live active lifestyles, and enjoy activity.

While interning at GE Medical Systems Corporate Fitness Center just outside Milwaukee, a few of my favorite coworkers asked me to train for a local 8-K in Milwaukee called AL'S Run. "How long is an 8-K?" I asked.

When I found out that it was just under 5 miles, I said, "I could never run that long!"

My friends gently guided me through 10 weeks of training. Every week I ran just a few steps farther than I had run the week before. Every week my friends would look me square in the eyes and repeat, "I told you so." "You CAN do this." "It's all in your head," they told me.

On a crisp fall morning in Milwaukee, I lined up for my first race. I didn't know what to expect. I didn't believe I would finish. I worried that if I finished at all, I would finish last. Despite my fear, I found the courage through friendship and camaraderie to try.

Well, I did finish. And I didn't finish last. As I crossed that finish line, I smiled for the cameras.

I went on to run longer, faster, and smarter. I found my inner long-distance athlete and ran my way through dozens of marathons. I even ran fast enough to qualify for the Boston

Marathon. Yes, that's right; I, the girl who came in *last* in gym class, qualified for the Boston Marathon, the most elite of marathons.

I began coaching runners and walkers in 1993. I created the training company called I Think I Can, and it was a home for adults wanting to train for and complete half- and full marathons.

Years later I was granted the opportunity to coach for the world's largest endurance training program, Team in Training (TNT). I began my journey with TNT in 1997 with the hopes of helping more people to reach the finish line and, more important, to find a cure for leukemia.

I eventually decided this is what I wanted to do with my life and joined forces with my friend Mike Norman to start Chicago Endurance Sports. CES is a company that trains new and seasoned walkers, runners, triathletes, and adventure racers.

You see, I am not a collegiate coach or an elite runner. I'm a mortal, just like you. I'm a woman who has learned through education, personal triumph, and many people's training stories, questions, and experiences how to make the transition from mere mortal to long-distance athlete.

How We Wrote This Book

Each chapter of *Marathoning for Mortals* begins with a question that we've been asked and is followed by an answer that is really a conversation between John and Jenny. You'll get to hear both of our voices. You'll get to read where we agree and where we don't. Think of us as the Click and Clack of the running world. You'll get two perspectives on every issue, every challenge, and every problem that you might encounter.

You'll come to see, we think, that in some cases there are no clear answers. Sometimes the answers are elusive even to those with years of training and experience. You'll also come to see that there are some unavoidable truths about being a long-distance athlete that the gifted and the less-than-gifted have to accept.

You'll learn that sometimes enthusiasm is your biggest asset, and at other times it is your greatest liability. You'll learn that sometimes less is more, and often less is plenty. You'll learn that your mind can trick your body and that your body is limited more by your imagination than by your biomechanics.

We'll be with you every step of the way with helpful hints from other runners and walkers and our own unique blend of solid coaching advice and Penguin philosophy. With a combination like that, your success is all but guaranteed.

Join us now on a journey where the finish line is just the beginning.

Part One

Getting Started

The most important step toward

success is getting to know yourself

CHAPTER ONE

Deciding to Train

The first step—deciding to train—transforms more mortals into adult-onset athletes than the last step across the finish line.

Mortal Dilemma: *I am an average recreational runner. I run just for the fun of it, to relieve stress, and to maintain my weight. Why should I decide to start training for a half- or full marathon?*

Entering my first race as a 43-year-old male created a turning point in my new life as an adult-onset athlete. I came from a motorsports racing background. I had watched lots of races and even took a few shots at racing everything from Grand Prix sidecars to the drag strip. For me, racing meant competition, beating your opponent, and walking away with trophies.

In my first running race, a 5-K/25-K/5-K duathlon, I really thought that I was going to compete to win. After all, I would be competing only against other men my age (at the time, age 43). I had already improved my speed dramatically; I had started at a 20-minute-per-mile pace and was down closer to a 10½-minute-per-mile pace.

I thought I'd be right up there with the leaders.

I even lined up in the front row. My first race ever, and I lined up in the front row! Lucky for me, a friend dragged me to the back of the pack, which was where I started . . . and finished.

I learned an important lesson that day. For nearly everyone out there, the race wasn't about competition, but rather about celebration. I couldn't believe how many of the other participants cheered for me as I struggled to cross that first finish line. They didn't make me feel as if I was a failure for finishing last. In fact, they made me feel as if I had just won an Olympic gold medal.

From that day on, my running and walking experience revolved around racing. I entered races as often as I could.

Since then, I've learned that there's a big difference between running for recreation and training for a specific event. The late George Sheehan once wrote, "The difference between a jogger and a runner is a race number." Few use the term *jogger* anymore, but his point still resonates. There is a huge difference between those who enjoy running as an activity and those who enjoy running as a sport.

Recreation vs. Sport

If you asked 1,000 people why they run or walk for recreation, you'd probably get nearly 1,000 different answers. The top reasons range from weight management and stress relief to quiet time alone and social time with friends.

If you make the transition from recreational running to training for a race, those 1,000 reasons then filter down to just a few. Whether you're in the front or the back of the pack, everyone trains for three—and only three—reasons.

1. You train to improve.
2. You train to maintain.
3. As you get older, you train to slow your rate of decline.

If you put your shoes on for any other reason, it's recreation. There's nothing magical about training to race, but racing does require you to change your focus from the nebulous and unseen benefits of reducing stress to the very specific, very easy-to-see results of running a faster mile.

Everything changes when you decide to train. Your goals change. Your life structure changes. Your risks change. Eventually, your rewards even change.

Let's start with your goals. If being active is your only goal (and that's a very worthy goal), then you don't need any more specifics. In fact, your goal can be intentionally unspecific. The goal of being more active may be the only goal you need.

If you switch over to training for a race, your goals become *very* specific. One of the ways you can help decide whether you are running or walking for recreation or training is by looking at just how specific your goals are. If you want to be able to run or walk a half- or full-marathon distance *some*day, then that's recreation. If you decide that you want to walk or run the Foot and Mouth Marathon in Spring Valley, Idaho, at 8 A.M. on November 5th and you want to finish it the same day you start. . . . now you've moved into training mode.

Not only do your big goals change when you decide to train, but so do your monthly, weekly, and even daily goals. You are no longer content to go out and just complete the miles. Every time you lace up your shoes, you know what your goal is, what your objectives are, and the outcome that you expect.

Now for the structure. To be successful at living an active life, you don't need structure. For the most part, you can be active on a regular basis, running or walking as far or as fast as you want, whenever you want. That's all the structure you need.

When you decide to train, your running and walking life becomes *very* structured. You have the long-term structure of your training program, the short-term structure of your training week, and the microstructure of your training day. You have particular workouts to complete at particular times. You must follow a particular diet. And you even must stick to a particular sleep schedule.

What used to pass for structure—say, getting out of the house three days a week—now seems like lifestyle anarchy.

Your risks also change when you move from recreation to racing. There aren't many risks for the recreational athlete. You should never be walking or running when you have an ache or pain.

When you move into training mode, you accept the risks of knowing that you will have to test your limits from time to time. You'll experience the limits of your body, the limits of your mind, and the limits of your spirit.

Many people think that only elite athletes find those limits and take those risks. That's wrong. All of us mortals do. Every one of us who takes on the challenge of going farther or faster is taking the same risk.

We all must find that edge between doing just enough to accomplish our goals and doing just a little too much and undermining our training. It is an edge—a very narrow line between doing what we must do and what we shouldn't do. And not many of us are very good at hitting that line every time.

The result is that often, in a training program, you feel as if you're somewhere between too much and not enough. You never feel quite settled about when to try to do a little more and when to do a little less. For us, that's part of the fun, knowing that at any minute we could have a break*through* or a break*down*.

Finally, the rewards intensify when you switch from running and walking for recreation to training for a race. The recreational rewards, as important as they are, are usually not the kinds of things that you can wrap your arms around. It may be great to lower your cholesterol by 50 points, but I don't know many people who walk around excited about it for a week.

In a training program, your reward is the race itself. On top of that, sometimes the racing spirits will reward you with a personal best, or the perfect day, or some other extraordinary experience that you will carry with you for the rest of your life.

We feel rewarded simply by getting out there on the racecourse and trying our best. You have to take whatever talent you have, train as well as you can, and then go out and see what happens. And it's true at the back of the pack as well as the front. Our reward is finding out for sure just what we have in us that day. It isn't always a faster time or a farther distance that brings us the reward. Sometimes it's simply knowing that we put it all together and gave it our best shot.

Mortal Questions, Honest Answers

Before you take the first step in your training program, you've got to make some decisions that will enable you to participate in the training.

You see, starting a training program is a little like finding your-self stranded on a deserted island. Whether you survive, whether you are successful, is mostly a matter of taking the time to look around and see what you have to work with. You must find what you have plenty of, what you're going to need, and what you can learn to do without.

Your first decision: Can you commit the time to training? Most of us don't have more time than we know what to do with. If you do, that's great. But most of us must carve our training time out of

Mortal Miracle

"If you lined up 100 people, I would have been the *last* one in that group you'd pick to run a marathon. I was a typical busy working woman, wife, mother, and community and church volunteer who could find time for everyone but herself. At least, that's what I told myself.

"When I was 40, a personal trainer helped me get on track to make some positive changes, including finishing a 5-K race. Still, the idea of a marathon sounded as impossible as climbing Mount Everest! Then, my friend Paige was diagnosed with leukemia. As I shared that difficult journey with her, Team in Training began organizing teams for the inaugural Country Music Marathon. In my zeal to do something positive to help Paige, I signed up.

"So how does a nonrunner and frequent fitness failure complete a marathon? For me, shifting the focus from myself to another person freed me from my own insecurities. As I concentrated on helping Paige, I found a new level of commitment and dedication to training.

"As I prepared for the marathon, every new milestone seemed like a miracle. At 6 miles, 12 seemed impossible. At 12 miles, 6 looked easy, but 18 seemed unreachable. On my final 21-mile training day, I knew I could complete the once inconceivable goal of 26.2 miles.

"The marathon was one of my top life experiences, ranking right up there with my wedding day and the births of my two children! I savored every step of the 26.2 miles, amazed at how far I'd come."

—Meryll, age 45

an already busy life. If that's the case for you, it doesn't make sense to start out thinking that you can handle a training program that requires more time than you can possibly commit. Pick one that fits your schedule.

Maybe you really want to run a marathon but your life is so busy that you can't find the time for the weekend long runs. (We'll get to those later. For now, just know that these runs build in time to 3 or more hours.) Okay, that should tell you that you're not ready to commit to running a full marathon. Rather, you should train for a half-marathon. It's far better to be successful at training for something that you can do than having to quit training because you weren't realistic about your time resources.

Other important questions follow from there. Knowing your answers—your honest answers—to these questions will help you firmly decide not only to train, but also to follow the right training plan for your body and goals.

Take a moment to think about the following:

◆ What other responsibilities do you have? Are you a single parent? How will you handle your child care? Are you a pet owner? Who's going to watch your pooch while you go out and do your long runs?

◆ What's your activity history? Have you been running or walking for years? Is this your first foray into the wonderful world of living an active, healthy lifestyle? Have you ever tried to train for a long-distance race in the past? If so, what happened? Did you complete the training? Did you finish the race? Did you feel good about the experience?

◆ What do you expect to get out of the training program? Do you want to run or walk in a particular event? Are you doing this really to experience the joys of running a marathon or because you want to lose weight and you think training will motivate you to change your eating habits?

◆ Are you training for yourself or someone else? Are you getting out there every day because it's what you want for yourself, or are you trying to prove something to someone?

◆ Are your expectations realistic? Are you willing—right now— to accept that getting to the starting line is your primary goal? Notice that I didn't say "finishing." I said "starting." Once the race starts, you must run and walk in the moment. Racing is a giant unknown. But getting to the starting line is something you can control.

◆ What else in your life could intervene and prevent you from getting to the starting line? What else in your life could take priority over your training? Who in your life is most likely to support you in this goal? Who is going to do everything possible to make it difficult for you?

Think carefully about these questions. They will help you later to thoughtfully pick the right training plan for your lifestyle, your body, and your goals. You can't simply pick a program at random and just start training. That's the worst thing you could do. You have to do the training—the real you, the you who has obligations and responsibilities, the you who has a life that you're already living that you now want to alter to accept the additional challenges of training.

The Mind-Body Connection

Beyond contemplating questions that address the physical you, you should also take some time to make some preliminary conclusions about the emotional you. Long-distance training can become an isolating and solitary pursuit if you're not careful. Are you the kind of person who wants and needs the time alone, or do you do best if you're in a group?

As the time and miles begin to add up, do you think you'll be happy to spend 2, 3, or 4 hours out on the roads by yourself? Or will you be better off finding others who are training so that you'll have company on your long runs?

Before you take the first step, it's also important to take a quick psychic inventory. No long-distance training program goes perfectly. It can't. For most runners and walkers, you are going up to and beyond your limits nearly every week. There will be workouts that bring you great satisfaction and workouts that will bring you to your knees in frustration.

Are you ready for that?

How well do you handle disappointment? How quickly do you recover from disappointment? As a long-distance athlete, you will have to learn to take the good and the bad in stride. You will have to learn to accept that not every run will be what you want it to be. You will have to learn to allow your body and your mind to adjust to the new stresses, the new strengths, and the new weaknesses. And you'll have to do it all while staying focused on the real goal: starting the race.

Long-distance training can be a positive and constructive form of selfishness. After all, once you're at the starting line, you're there by yourself. No one can run a single step for you. No one can jump in and help you. No one but you can make the decisions about what to do to keep going. It's all up to you.

Honesty Is the Best Marathon Policy

The biggest mistake most new long-distance athletes make is overestimating their level of readiness. Too often, people begin a training program based more on the miles they wish they had gotten in than the miles they actually ran or walked.

There's no advantage to your doing that with any of the *Marathoning for Mortals* programs. Based on your answers to the questions in this chapter as well as to the personal inventory in chapter 3, and based on *your* goals and *your* life, you'll be able to choose a program that will all but guarantee your success. And choosing a program today doesn't mean that you'll have to stick with that program forever. You can move up, down, and around the various programs as you see how your body reacts to the training stresses and how well you can hold off the rest of your life as you train.

This is the time to get very, *very* honest with yourself. It's easy enough to say that you want to run a marathon in under 4 hours in just 4 months of training, but wishing and wanting won't make it so. It's easy enough to say you want to walk a half-marathon in under 4 hours in just 4 months, but that is no easier a goal to reach depending on where you are right now.

How do you decide whether you're being too ambitious or setting your goals too low? You can't really tell until you start training. Just be prepared to switch to a program that both suits your needs and fits into your lifestyle at any time. Don't allow yourself to feel like you must stay with the program that you first pick.

Robert Pirsig wrote that mountains should be climbed at a pace in between exhaustion and boredom. If you climb too slowly, you find yourself getting bored with the pace and the activity. If you climb too quickly, you find yourself so winded that you can't enjoy the beauty of the experience. The same is true for your training program. You should find the place in between boredom and exhaustion.

Long-distance training is, by definition, the process of going a little farther and reaching a little deeper just about every week. Your long training sessions, as they begin to move upward on the mileage scale, will require more mental, physical, and emotional stamina than you have right now. That's the good news.

If you find that you are making every excuse possible to avoid the long training sessions, you need to figure out why. And, back to Pirsig, chances are that you're going either too fast or too slow. The avoidance is the same, but the symptoms are different.

If you train at a pace that is slower than your optimum pace, you'll begin to feel as if you're just not getting anywhere. The time will seem to go by at a snail's pace. You'll find yourself looking at your watch every few minutes, disheartened because it'll seem like you're standing still.

If you train at a pace that is too fast, you'll find yourself hating life, hating running, and looking at the watch and feeling like it's moving backward. You won't understand why you are working so hard and yet the watch doesn't reward you with the passage of time.

So when you decide to train, choose your program, and make your training plan, be sure to find the one that is best for you. It may not be possible for all of your friends to share your training plan. It may not be possible for you to share theirs. That's the beauty of it all. You can choose *your* plan. They can choose *their* plan. When it's over, you can show each other the medals you won!

Know Before You Go

Before turning to chapter 2, reread the questions in the last part of this chapter. Promise that you will be honest to yourself, your body, and your training. Only you can put in the miles and run the race. Remember:

- Long-distance athletes are made, not born.
- Racing can add spice to your walking and running life.

■ Training to do your best is the purest form of competition.

■ There's a difference between recreation and racing.

■ Knowing where you want to go begins with knowing where you arc.

■ The best program is the program that is best for *you*.

■ No one knows you better than you know yourself.

■ If at first you don't succeed, try a different program.

■ Goals can never be too high, but expectations can.

CHAPTER TWO

Who, Where, When, and Why

Think of a long-distance athlete. Do you see a solitary individual logging in lonely miles along some forgotten highway? Well, it isn't that way anymore. For proof, just hang out at a half- or full-marathon finish and see for yourself who is out there running, walking, and waddling across the finish line.

Mortal Dilemma: *Can I really finish a long-distance race? I have never raced, and I am not a typical runner or fast walker.*

Marathoning is no longer reserved for the mechanically efficient. All mortals who are willing to take that first step to train, prepare, and show up can participate in the marathon. Thousands of adult-onset athletes train every year. And thousands finish.

So, can you do it? The answer to that question lies hidden beneath your fears. The true question is this: Are you willing to take the time to train, prepare, and change your lifestyle? There is no such thing as a typical runner or walker anymore. Mortals just like you are "doing it" every season, every race, every day.

For most new long-distance athletes, the odyssey starts with a fearful question and turns into a life-changing, eye-opening journey. At the start of every TNT training program, people ask Jenny whether she thinks they can actually complete the race. She always answers "Yes." In her experience, once any mortal makes the decision to begin training, the evolution begins, from purchasing the right shoes to altering social plans to actually putting one foot in front of the other.

—⟋⟍—

Like Coach Jenny, I love long-distance races. I didn't always. At first I couldn't understand why anyone would want to put him- or herself through what looked like untold torture. That was a long time ago, long before I ever accepted the challenge of trying to cover a distance on foot that I used to feel bored to drive in a car.

Now, for me, there's nothing like the feeling of lining up at the starting line with a few thousand of my closest friends with nothing to do that day except make my way to the finish line. I can stand there and know that thousands of folks just like me, who share my values and goals, are—for the most part—going in the same direction as I am.

It's not that I have a gift for the distance. I don't. Runners like Khalid Khannouchi and Paula Radcliffe have a gift for the distance. I was lucky enough, twice, to witness both of them winning a marathon. Khalid won with cunning and an elegant strategy; Paula won with a display of sheer courage and determination.

Heck, I don't even have any talent for the distance. I've known folks who started running and walking well into their fifties and sixties who've discovered a mother lode of talent that they never dreamed they had. These are the people who show up at their first marathon, run a Boston qualifying time, and tell you later that they didn't even know they had to qualify to run the Boston marathon.

After years of running, walking, and observing the longer-distance races, I've learned that true long-distance success is more about tenacity than talent. The successful new long-distance athlete is the one who can leave his or her ego behind at the race's start. And the successful veteran long-distance athlete is the one who knows that the mystery of the distance can never be fully solved.

Nearly anyone who is willing to take the time to carefully prepare can go the distance. Anyone, even a mortal like you, who is willing to carve the time out of his or her life and commit to a training program can go the distance.

In fact, the longer the distance, the more the miles will forgive you for not having a gift or talent and will reward you for your

Mortal Miracle

"I've been running for 4 years. During that time, I've run two half-marathons. Both times, when I crossed the finish line, I felt rewarded for the hard work that went into my training. I walked away knowing that I could accomplish anything. That positive attitude has led me to finish three triathlons as well. Now, I'm training for the Myrtle Beach Marathon, a distance that deserves respect. You don't have to be a professional athlete to achieve great things. Even an unknown 10-minute miler, like me, can bask in the glory of race day success."

—Pam, age 33

tenacity and preparation. I can't give you any hard science to prove that, but I offer as evidence the smiles of the thousands of ordinary people just like us who finish long-distance races every weekend.

One thing is certain: More people are participating in long-distance races, and they are taking their time and enjoying them more. My first complete marathon was in Columbus, Ohio, in 1993. I finished in just under 5 hours. And I was nearly dead last.

Recently, I finished the Suzuki Rock 'n' Roll marathon in 5 hours and 40 minutes, and there were nearly 8,000 people behind me. In fact, if I can convince enough people to run the long-distance races more slowly than I do, I might make it to the middle of the pack!

I can guarantee that back where I start, you'll see people of every shape and size, age, gender, and economic stratum. You'll find people running their first marathon and their 100th. You'll talk to the woman who got sick of the old man and threw him out, joined a marathon training program, and is participating as a way of celebrating her new life.

Of course, what she doesn't realize is that the guy she threw out quit smoking and drinking, lost 35 pounds, and is standing just a few yards away.

Why

If you asked 1,000 participants why they decided to run longer races, you'd get 1,000 answers. There may be some common answers, but if you dig a little deeper, you'll almost always find a personal reason why someone takes the challenge.

The challenge of the distance draws people in thousands. I tell people all the time that if completing a half- or full marathon were easy, everyone would be out there doing it. Some of us train to get away from the realities of our lives. Some of us train to prove to our inner demons that we can do it. Some of us train to find our limits.

—∿—

I, Jenny, remember finishing my first half-marathon at the Lake County Races in early spring 1992. Those races officially kicked off the racing season in the Chicago area. The course was unique. Rather than traveling in a circle, the course reached from one point to another and included a 10-K, half-marathon, and full marathon. All three races shared the same starting line. The finish for each race was at a different location. Every participant, fast or slow, got a good taste of reality pie from the very beginning with a train ride 26.2 miles from the marathon finish line to the start. Every minute the train moved north, we saw yet another mile we would have to run or walk.

I finished that first half-marathon not a minute too soon. I don't think I could have run another step. I'm glad I found the finish line when I did, or things would have gotten ugly quickly. I gathered up the postrace goodies and my finisher's medal and stepped up onto the train to ride back to the marathon finish and my car. (By the way, stepping up stairs after a race is an evil thing. I think every muscle in my body ached. Asking my body to lift itself up stairs was like overtime—painful but necessary.)

The train took off south to the finish and followed the marathon course along the way. As I watched those runners at the 15th, 18th, 20th, and 24th miles, I kept thinking that there was no way—no way—I could have ever kept running. The thought of going *another* 13.1 miles felt impossible at the time, out of my mental reach.

Like childbirth, the pain of running clears and makes way for exciting race stories and many prideful occasions to wear your race shirt. It was not much later when a little voice began to speak, telling me to run a full marathon. "Come on," said the little voice. "You really didn't feel all that bad at the half-marathon finish. After all, if you can finish a half, why can't you finish a full marathon?"

And so it went—the half-marathon success got put in a box of past successes and a new goal emerged.

I finished my first marathon in Chicago. I felt surprised, shocked, and overwhelmed. I earned the soreness, the medal, and the glory. And a few days later, I heard the little voice telling me to train to qualify for Boston. I had gone from trying to make it down my block to running 26.2 miles.

The distances are relative to what you know and what you are willing to accomplish. I pushed myself to find my limits, to prove to myself and others that I can reach my dreams, and to quiet the demons that kept me and my fears hostage for years.

Not all the whys are elaborate answers like mine. Your why might be pretty simple. It might just be something you've always wanted to do. It might be that you have a friend, spouse, or family member who has run one.

Conversely, the whys can get more complicated. Spend any time with the participants who are part of one of the charity programs (such as the Leukemia and Lymphoma Society's Team in Training) and you will find stories of hope, stories of loss, and stories of overcoming the odds.

—〰—

I once ran with a woman who was finishing a marathon to celebrate her life. She had survived a double organ transplant. Did she care about her time? No way. Every minute of her life was already a gift—and she knew it.

Your why may also be a matter of principle or a matter of honor. My then-27-year-old son ran a marathon with me because he couldn't admit that his then-50-year-old father could do something he couldn't do. Even though he paid the price of not training, he still experienced the satisfaction of finishing.

There is no right answer to why. There is no wrong answer, either.

Where

People often ask me, John, to name my favorite marathon. I try to explain that it's like asking the parents of 10 kids to name their favorite child. As with all children, all marathons are unique and special.

Yet, for your first marathon, I suggest you pick a location that offers the following characteristics.

- Plenty of people cheering on the sidelines
- Lots of volunteer support at the aid stations and all along the course
- A generous finish-line closing time (at least 6 hours for run/walkers and 8 hours for walkers) so that you don't have any anxiety about finishing in time to get a medal

For a half-marathon, the same holds true. You need to make sure that you choose an event that understands that your main goal is to have a good time, not to finish with a fast time. Of course, if you finish with a fast time, then you probably had a fantastic time, but I digress.

I'll admit that I'm partial to big-city marathons. I'm a city kid. I like the asphalt. I like the concrete and steel. I like the energy that comes from running and walking through a major urban area. I admire any city that allows thousands of people to see it from ground level.

The LaSalle Bank Chicago Marathon is one of my favorites, mostly because it's where I grew up and still live. There's something special about running around the streets of home and seeing the city for the first time as an athlete in the company of other athletes.

—ww—

I agree with John to a certain extent. The LaSalle Bank Chicago Marathon is also one of my favorites. I get a rush running through hometown streets. We, the marathoners, own the city for a day. I know exactly where I am during every mile. There is nothing like finishing among the buildings and people in my hometown. The race is a celebration for the whole city, not just the participants.

But as much as I enjoy the Chicago marathon, I actually prefer to run races in the great outdoors, races that wind through scenic pathways with the sounds of nature cheering you on. Such races attract fewer participants but offer more to see along the way. I've seen deer while running a local half-marathon in a forest preserve, snakes in the wilds of the Southwest, and even a moose in the Mayor's Midnight Sun Marathon in Anchorage, Alaska. Rural races draw my primal strengths and push me like the winds.

Everyone is different and every course offers something for everyone. One of the greatest benefits to racing is being able to run and walk through the trails and streets of cities all over the world. It is almost as if every city opens up its streets just for you to experience. Running a marathon perhaps offers the very best way to get to know the culture, sights, and people of a city.

Mortal Miracle

"Why am I running a marathon? I ask myself that question every day, and every day I find a different answer.

"It's about:

◆ Setting goals and achieving them.

◆ Getting to know a running friend all over again.

◆ Hitting a wall and then learning to climb it.

◆ Knowing every inch of my body and responding to its every need.

◆ Mind over matter.

◆ Satisfaction at the end of the day.

◆ Smiling at mile 20.

"Above all, it's mental. I endured so much in those weeks of training. It made me the strongest I can be mentally. That's the most important power in my life. It has made me who I am. I've learned training for a marathon is more than just running—way more."

–Kelly, no age given

Every runner has unique interests. You'll find a race that fills your unique interests with sights and sounds to remember for a lifetime. Just identify what interests you and then sign up!

That may be fine for Coach Jenny, but not for me. It's not that I don't like the rural races; I do. It's just that the idea of running and walking for 6 hours with nothing to look at but twigs and branches just isn't my cup of tea. I know; I know. I've tried. It just isn't in me.

I ran the Wineglass Marathon in the fall in upstate New York, arguably one of the most beautiful marathons in the eastern United States. All around me, runners were raving about the trees, the burning red maples, and the flaming orange oaks. They waxed poetic about the glory of the leaves turning and the cycle of life that it implies.

I watched the road 20 feet in front of me. I am way too clumsy to spend a marathon looking around at trees and flowers that are a half-mile away. I might see a bouquet of roses if someone handed them to me, but I'd probably miss them out on the course.

When

Although we differ as to where we choose to complete marathons and half-marathons, we agree as to when to register for a race. It is easy to gather up the motivation to register at any time. However, come race day, you'd much rather be fully trained and injury-free than aching and half-prepared because you didn't give yourself enough time to train.

We've seen it all too often. People are lured into registering for a race at Walt Disney World or in Hawaii, but they don't have the time to train properly to get to the finish line. Once the race bug bites you, it is easy to get caught up in signing up for races prematurely. This almost always ends in an injury.

For any long-distance training program, you want to show up race-ready, properly trained, adequately rested, and fully nourished. For this to happen, you need time—time to build miles, time to rest and recover, and time to taper. Long-distance training is very demanding on the body and requires a sound mileage base from the beginning. Just like building a home, you can't paint the walls until you've drywalled them.

We've met more than our share of potential marathoners who can't muster the patience needed to build miles before attempting a long-distance race. Instead, they want to go from running their first miles ever to signing up for a marathon next month. It is true. We've met these people. We meet most of them somewhere on the marathon course. They're the ones hobbled over, crying, trying to remember why they started running this race.

Our training programs range from 14 weeks for the half-marathon to 20 weeks for the full marathon. However, if you've never run a step in your life, that doesn't mean you'll be ready to complete your marathon 4 or 5 months from today. As you read this book, you will discover that the length of your journey depends on where you are right now.

If you are already running or walking on a regular basis and simply want to add the half- or full-marathon training program to your schedule, you'll be able to do that. If you are just thinking about starting to become more active, you'll learn how to assess where you are and where you need to be before you take on the challenge of a long-distance training program. Rather than aiming for a full marathon, you might start with the 14-week half-marathon schedule. Once you finish your half, then you might consider the 20-week marathon schedule.

Start at the beginning and enjoy the journey. Enjoy the triumphs with shorter distances. Then over time, build the minutes, the miles, and the stories.

Can you be a long-distance athlete? Of course you can. We believe that with patience and determination you can change your life. And we believe that because we've both walked that road ahead of you.

Know Before You Go

Before you move on to chapter 3, take a moment to think about why *you* want to become a long-distance athlete. Know that you can complete the distance, as long as you have the courage to start and the patience to master each step along the way. Tentatively pick a date in the future by which you think you'd like to complete your first race. Do some research on half- and full marathons, finding one that meets your personal needs. But don't sign up just yet. After reading the next few chapters and choosing your training plan, you'll get a better idea of how long it will really take you to train.

Remember:

- Everyone can be a long-distance athlete.
- There is no such thing as the typical long-distance athlete.
- Someone in worse shape than you is already training.
- Deciding to train comes before preparing to train.
- There are different events that appeal to different people. Choose yours.
- Every race at every distance has unique challenges.
- Knowing why is as critical as knowing where you want to compete.
- Patience is your most important training tool.
- Tenacity is as essential as talent.
- There are no easy marathon courses.

CHAPTER THREE

Getting to Know You

Think you don't have the body of a long-distance athlete? Think there's something special about the way their bodies work? You're in for a surprise. There's less difference between them and you than you thought.

Mortal Dilemma: *I'd like to run a long-distance race, but I just don't feel like I have the right body for it. Is there a long-distance body?*

Even as a young boy, I didn't think I had an athlete's body. My legs were too short, my arms were too long, my butt was too big . . . well, you get the idea. I found every excuse to avoid activity. After all, if I didn't have the body for it, no one could expect me to even try.

Later, as I began to run and walk a little, and then a lot, I had to reevaluate my thinking. I could no longer ignore the evidence that I was, indeed, a runner. I could no longer discount the details that painted me as an athlete. To avoid accepting myself as a runner, I told myself that *real* runners ran long distances, and I didn't.

Then I ran and walked my first marathon.

It turns out, as I learned during my first marathon, that I do have the body of a long-distance athlete. So do you. In fact, every body can be the body of a long-distance athlete. No one's legs are too short. No one's arms are too long. And I can assure you that no one's butt is too big. Every body is a long-distance body.

Whether you're the world's record holder or a first-timer, you've got exactly the same physiology. The first runner to break the tape, the last runner to cross the finish, and every runner in between all usually have two feet and two legs, 206 bones, a heart, more than 600 muscles, and a brain.

Record holders don't have extra lungs or hearts. They don't have third legs that make them faster. Nope, as hard as it is to imagine, our bodies are the same as theirs.

Our bodies' systems are all the same. We've all got the same cardiovascular systems, the same respiratory systems, and the same musculoskeletal systems. Okay, they may not be *exactly* the same. I ran near Bill Rodgers once and understood immediately why he won the Boston Marathon four times and I didn't. He ran with grace, each footstrike propelling him forward like a gazelle. I ran with the waddling clumsiness of a—well—penguin. But he was still running with his own two feet, just like me.

To help you believe that you really do possess the body needed to become a long-distance athlete, let's take a look at the body systems that every long-distance athlete needs to succeed—just to make sure that you've got all the right parts in place.

The Heart of a Long-Distance Athlete

Let's start with the aerobic or cardiovascular system. This includes your heart, lungs, and blood vessels that carry all that wonderful oxygen to your muscles. We don't think much about this system because it works pretty well all by itself. You don't have to spend time during the day making sure that your heart is pumping and your lungs are sucking air.

So now that you've determined that you are, in fact, breathing, you've successfully passed the first test to determine whether you have the body of a long-distance athlete. Let's move on to the second test.

The Muscles of a Long-Distance Athlete

Your muscles are intricate creations made up of lots of fibers. You have your long and short fibers, your thick and thin fibers, and your strong and weak fibers. Some muscles are no longer than your finger. Others, like your hamstrings, go on forever. But no matter how long or short, they all respond the same way. They get stronger through the repetition of stress and recovery.

Mortal Miracle

"I've run five half-marathons and one marathon. I'm now training for my second marathon in Chicago. I am neither a fast runner nor a 'skinny runner.' (Trust me, I *never* will be either one!) The ability to run a half- or full marathon—and talk the whole time—has convinced me that I am truly a fit person. For me, it's not necessarily about running the marathon in a record time. It's about starting and finishing the race, knowing that I am in great shape. I can say, 'Look at me—I just ran 26.2 miles!'"

—Marlene, age 37

Think of muscles as a group of workers all sitting around waiting to be called into action. Most of the time, a small group of worker-fibers do all of the work. This group handles all the routine activities of life, such as walking around and brushing your teeth. If left alone, the other workers never have to get out of their chairs.

In an emergency—real or imagined—these extra workers show up for work, but they are not all that happy about it. If you've ever gone out and done something like pull weeds or play soccer for an afternoon, you know exactly what I'm talking about. Your muscles end up very sore due to the new activity.

As a long-distance athlete, you need to gently convince all those long-underused muscles that you really need their help. They'll co-operate if you bring them along slowly. Try to rush them and you're asking for trouble and *very* sore muscles. Everyone's muscles respond to exercise this way. The only difference between a nonath-lete's muscles and an athlete's muscles is that the athlete knows the right formula for getting muscles to respond to training.

Here's how most "get into shape in a week" programs work for nonathletes. On Monday, you go out and fatigue all those great muscles that have been carrying the load for most of your life. On Tuesday, when you go out to exercise again, the strong muscles are already tired, so they turn the work over to the less well prepared muscles nearby. Those muscles, of course, get fatigued much more quickly than the Monday muscles, so you get tired more easily.

On Wednesday, you're tired and achy. You've convinced your-self that you need discipline—and not rest—to succeed, so you ex-ercise *again*. Now the Monday muscles are shot, the Tuesday muscles don't even want to think about moving, and the Wednesday muscles have been so far from the action that they im-mediately organize a strike.

Thursday? Disaster day. You push your Monday-through-

Wednesday muscles into action one more time. The Thursday muscles, seeing the other muscles quickly display the surrender flag, give up immediately.

By Friday, your friends are asking why you're walking so funny, and you've convinced yourself that you just don't have an athlete's body. You go back to the old sedentary lifestyle, content that exercise just won't work for you.

Of course it doesn't have to happen that way. We mortals all have the potential to become athletes. We need only treat our muscles properly.

Here's the secret: If you give your muscles time to recover, they will come back stronger and more willing to go to work. If you get those Monday muscles working for you, the Tuesday muscles get excited and want in on the fun. Pretty soon, you've got Wednesday and Thursday involved, too, and the next thing you know, you're running and walking farther than you ever thought possible.

The Bones of a Long-Distance Athlete

Your skeletal system is the most delicate of all the body systems. It relies on your brain to keep your muscles from doing something stupid, such as wearing themselves out so much that the muscles can't hold the joints in place—something stupid like, oh, running or walking too far or too fast or too soon, adding mileage more quickly than your muscles can handle, or simply doing anything for too long.

If your brain doesn't keep your muscles from embarking on such stupid antics, your bones and joints respond with a painful series of sharp stabs and dull aches.

How do I know this? Because I spent the first 6 months of my running career limping around on swollen knees. I pulled myself up stairs and walked down steps backward. Sadly, I thought that the discomfort was the price I had to pay to be an athlete. I was wrong!

I had an athlete's body. But I was treating my body like a moron.

Treat your body like the body of an athlete, and your body will respond and grow into the body of an athlete. Becoming a long-distance athlete can be the journey of a lifetime. It will reward your patience. It will forgive your indiscretions as long as you don't push your luck. It will allow you to find paths to yourself that you didn't know were there.

Most important, with just a little bit of care and planning, you'll discover the biggest secret that your body holds—that you *do* have the body of a long-distance athlete.

The Training of a Long-Distance Athlete

Not long after I met John at running camp, we set up a time to run together. I was shocked to notice the funny walk and running gait he sported during the entire workout. It was almost as if his hip were duct-taped to his ribs on the right and his ear were taped to his shoulder on the left. He walked with a limp and ran with an uneven stride.

A few miles into the workout, he told me that he maintained his running lifestyle with hundreds of miles and tons of ibuprofen. It wasn't long before I launched into my coach's lecture, a lecture that I repeat often even to this day—to John and numerous other runners who seem to rank ibuprofen right up there with running shoes on their lists of essential running must-haves.

You see, sometimes our motivation to push ourselves forward becomes greater than our bodies can handle. When you push too hard and rest too little, injuries crop up. Life becomes less about reaching personal bests and more about rehabbing injuries.

It doesn't have to happen this way.

Only the smartest runners and walkers figure this out from the beginning. Training should be more about listening to your body and less about following a program to the exact mile or minute. A smart runner or walker listens closely and continually modifies the training plan to allow for adequate recovery. With the patience to recover, you can then push forward. Although patience is perhaps one of the hardest virtues to master, it makes the difference between showing up on race day in optimal condition and not showing up at all.

Training adaptation actually occurs while we rest. When we train, we break down our systems by placing them under stress. With rest, our bodies rejuvenate and grow stronger than the day before.

Without rest, our bodies remain stressed and eventually weaken due to lack of proper healing time.

When you push your body past its normal activity, it requires rest to adapt. In fact, it's during sleep that your body secretes the highest amounts of growth hormone, the hormone

Mortal Miracle

"Running has transformed my life. For the first 30 years of my life I weighed 250 pounds and wore a size 45. I was extremely shy and totally sedentary. During the past 8 years, I have run 20 marathons, more than ten 50-K trail runs, two 50-milers, and a 100-K race. I now weigh 185 pounds!"

—Grant, age 38

responsible for healing and strengthening your muscles. Give your body rest and it will adapt, grow stronger, and—as if by magic—be able to run or walk longer and faster. Rob your body of rest and you'll grow weaker, run more slowly, and eventually get sick and injured.

So remember the optimal formula for success: Work hard, rest, work hard, rest. Also, keep in mind the optimal formula for disaster: Work hard, work hard, work hard.

Your Personal Inventory

Starting a training program requires you to take a personal inventory of what you have and what you will need to pack on this journey. It requires getting to know yourself and assessing your assets and liabilities. It requires taking an honest look at how old you are, how often you move, and how many dings and dents you've acquired through the years.

You should follow the training program that makes the most sense for you. There is no one magic training program to satisfy everyone's needs. Sure, you can follow any random program out there in the virtual world, but will it push you to an injury or not even prepare you at all? How do you know it will match your health history, exercise history, and goals?

The smartest way to begin a long-distance program is to stop and take a long, hard look inside. Where are you now? Where do you want to go? What do you have to work with? What needs a little work? These questions will help you personalize your program to meet your needs and expectations.

So to find the perfect training plan for your body, let's sit down together and get to know you a little better.

We created the following questions to help you gather personal information about your past, present, and future. Try to answer these questions honestly and thoroughly. The more honest you are now, the better your training will progress later. You will use your answers here to pinpoint the best training plan for you of the eight different *Marathoning for Mortals* programs that we've included at the end of the book, starting on page 224.

We recommend writing the questions and answers down on a separate piece of paper. Tuck that piece of paper securely between the pages of *Marathoning for Mortals*. We'll ask you to refer to it often as you progress along your journey. Also, from time to time, we'll ask you to go back to your answers to make sure that the course you've chosen is the course you still want to be on.

You can use this personal inventory season after season to help you decide over and over which program makes the most sense for you at that particular time. Let's do it.

What is your age?

A. *18–30*
B. *31–40*
C. *41–50*
D. *51+*

What is your gender?

A. *Female*
B. *Male*
C. *Superhuman android*

What is your weight?

A. *My weight is appropriate for my height, and I don't consider myself overweight.*
B. *I am less than 10 pounds over my ideal weight.*

C. *I am 10–25 pounds over my ideal weight.*

D. *I am 26–50 pounds over my ideal weight.*

E. *I am 51+ pounds over my ideal weight.*

Describe your general health.

A. *I have never had any health problems.*

B. *I have been under a doctor's care for ailments, but I am currently healthy.*

C. *I am under a doctor's care for a chronic medical condition.*

D. *I will be lucky to get to the end of the day.*

Describe your injury history.

A. *I have never had an injury in my life.*

B. *I have had injuries, but they have since healed, and I am currently injury-free.*

C. *I am currently (or should be) under a doctor's care for an injury.*

D. *I am in complete denial about my injuries even though I can barely walk.*

Describe your current activity level.

A. *I participate in some form of continuous aerobic activity most days of the week (4–6 days).*

B. *I participate in some form of continuous aerobic activity some days of the week (1–3 days).*

C. *I have participated in continuous aerobic activity, but never consistently.*

D. *Opening this book is the most exercise I've had in 6 months.*

Describe your past activity level.

A. *I have been active for more than one year.*

B. *I have been active for more than 6 months.*

C. *I have been active for a few months.*

D. *I have been active for a few minutes.*

What is your training goal?

A. *I would like to finish the race.*

B. *I would like to finish in a particular time goal.*

C. *I have already completed the distance and would like to improve my finish time.*

D. *I would just like to finish reading this book.*

How many days per week can you commit to training?

A. *5 days per week*

B. *3–4 days per week*

C. *2–3 days per week*

How much time can you commit to training?

A. *8–10 hours per week*

B. *6–8 hours per week*

C. *4–6 hours per week*

List the top three factors that motivate you to exercise (e.g., lose weight, train with a group, follow a structured program, relieve stress, find time for myself, have a goal to reach for).

1.

2.

3.

List your top three challenges to finishing this training program (e.g., lack of time, lack of motivation, lack of support).

1.

2.

3.

If you've answered the questions honestly, you already have a head start on most participants in long-distance training programs. Honesty is always the best policy, and for a long-distance athlete, even a little dishonesty at mile 1 of the training program can lead to disaster somewhere down the road.

When you're ready, turn to chapter 4 and let's start making the plan.

Know Before You Go

You have everything you need to become a long-distance athlete. You have the feet, the legs, the heart, and the mind. Once you embark on the right training plan for your body and fitness background, you'll have taken a huge step toward marathon success.

Before moving on to chapter 4, make sure you have completed your personal inventory. Without those answers, you will lack the map needed to guide your training.

Remember:

- You have to train the body you have.
- Elite athletes' bodies have the same systems as ours.
- Every body responds to training.
- Who you can be doesn't depend on who you have been.
- Choose a training program that fits you.
- Be honest about your abilities, goals, and dreams.
- Pain is like an annoying friend. Ignoring it won't make it go away.
- Train your body like your favorite pet, with kindness and love.
- Even if today is day 1, tomorrow will be day 2.
- The most difficult road is the road to understanding.

CHAPTER FOUR

Making the Plan

Getting to where you want to go starts with knowing where you are. Only then can you match where you are to the training program that will take you where you want to go.

Mortal Dilemma: *How do I know which training program is best for me?*

We can't assign a one-size-fits-all training program to everyone who reads this book. But we can guide you in making the right decision by helping you to choose the right training program for you.

We've included eight different training programs in the appendix of *Marathoning for Mortals*. Each plan prepares you for a different goal, ranging from walking a half-marathon to running an entire marathon. To achieve each goal, you'll follow a different journey, one that will prepare your body, mind, and soul for race day.

Yet, as with many college courses, some of our training plans require *previous* training. Others do not. You must first pick the right goal for your body at this particular time—and then follow the plan that will help you meet that goal.

Back to That Personal Inventory

To help ensure that you start off with wisdom and patience as well as that you reach for the right goal and pick the best training plan for you, let's take look at a fictional participant's personal inventory. The details that follow will help you to better examine your answers to your personal inventory—allowing you to start your marathon journey on the right foot.

What is your age?

Jane B. Fit: I am 39 years old.

As we age, our bodies need more time to recover. Because aches and pains take longer to heal, an older runner such as Jane needs a program that includes more rest in between training sessions.

Imagine a pyramid of life. The incline of the pyramid represents years 1 to 30 and the decline illustrates years 31 and onward. On one side we are improving continually, while on the other we are declining slowly. We're not trying to depress you, but rather to explain why your age affects the best training program for you.

Distance athletes in their twenties can get away with a lot more mileage and a lot less rest. Their bodies are more resilient and bounce back quickly. Once we hit our thirties, our bodies need a little more tender loving care to get through workouts and prepare for races. With youth we have energy and vitality, but with age comes the wisdom to train smart and listen to the body.

What is your gender?

Jane B. Fit: Female

When it comes to gender there are, well, a few differences.

To see the difference between the strengths of men and women, look at the difference in finishing times for a 5-K, then a marathon, and then a 100-mile ultra. (Yes, people really do run that far in one shot!) Though no woman has come close to beating a man at the 5-K or marathon distance, Ann Trason has won the overall category in ultra marathons numerous times—beating the women *and* the men. So we all have our strengths; we just need to learn how to tap into them and use them to benefit our performance.

Guys, know from the very beginning that you can run fast. But it is not always wise to come in first. Your bodies need to acquire the mileage base to support this urge. Ladies, know that you can run for miles and burn lots of calories, but doing so without a mileage base will not necessarily drop the pounds like you may think and just may push you to burnout or injury.

Of course, gender is not the most important factor in your training. Age, general health, overall level of fitness, and lifestyle mean much more. Whether male or female, be smart, be patient, and learn to use your strength and endurance to benefit your program.

What is your weight?

Jane B. Fit: I am 25–50 pounds over my ideal weight.

Jane will be carrying extra weight while training, and this extra weight will create more impact on her muscles and joints with every footstrike as she runs or walks.

She can reduce some of her extra weight by training at the right intensity and frequency. This same tactic will also allow her to run or walk more efficiently eventually. Jane will need to start with a conservative program that includes walking and builds gradually to run/walking. This approach will teach her body how to adapt to impact and ultimately allow her to progress readily, without injuries. Her patience will have to take precedence over her motivation to run.

Describe your general health.

Jane B. Fit: I have been under a doctor's care for ailments, but I am currently healthy.

Jane had a baby more than 3 years ago and was under the care of a doctor for the duration of the pregnancy. Although she has recovered, she still struggles with losing the weight she gained during the pregnancy. Therefore, her pregnancy, although in the past, is still a factor today.

Like Jane B. Fit, your health—past or present—is an important factor when considering training programs. Consider all health ailments such as diabetes, knee pain, low back pain, or even heart conditions before starting the training process. We highly recommend that you advise your doctor about your goal to train for a half- or full marathon. Take the time to review your current health and discuss your past with your doctor. Your doctor can give you specific tips or modifications to aid your training program.

Describe your injury history.

Jane B. Fit: I have had injuries, but they have since healed, and I am currently injury-free.

Jane, after having her baby, decided to begin running to lose weight. Three weeks into her program, she developed pain in the bottom of her right foot. She was diagnosed with plantar fasciitis (one of the top three running injuries that you will learn more about in chapter 9). She was told to rest and ice her foot frequently. She got discouraged and hasn't run since.

There are a couple things at play here. For some people, running too soon drastically increases the likelihood of an injury early

Mortal Miracle

"Running my first marathon at age 32 was an incredible experience. My father had multiple sclerosis, and at age 32 he was walking with crutches. My father has since passed away. I felt as if he were with me the entire race. My memories of him helped me through both the race and the intense training leading up to it. I never walked at all during the marathon, even though the last few miles were very difficult and emotional. I felt like my dad had helped me along. Thanks, Dad."

—Brian, age 37

in the game. Jane's body was not ready for the impact. She had never run before. She had never even walked for fitness before. She was also carrying more weight than normal. Her body simply raised the red flag to warn her that she was headed down the wrong path.

As we mentioned earlier, Jane should have started with a walking program to get her body used to the impact. Then she could progress to running without the resulting foot pain.

Your past or present aches, pains, or even injuries offer important clues to the best training program for you. They will also help you listen vigilantly to your body. Your body has a wonderful memory. Chances are that the spots where you hurt in the past are the same spots where you will hurt in the future. Listening to such discomfort and modifying your training before a minor ache or pain turns into a major injury will help you stay on track.

A past injury won't keep you from completing one of the training programs. A past injury doesn't mean that you can never be a long-distance athlete. It does mean that you need to be aware of what contributed to the injury in the past and make sure that you avoid doing those things again. Take care of your body. It is the only one you have to work with.

Describe your current and past activity levels.

Jane B. Fit: I have participated in continuous aerobic activity, but never consistently.

Jane has tried almost everything, but never for very long. She walked, ran, and participated in step, boxing, and even judo classes. She wants to stick with a program and succeed.

Identifying your trend in activity level determines what you have or have not been doing. Like Jane, if you haven't been active in months and have struggled with staying consistent every week, then it makes the most sense to start with a program that gradually incorporates training into your lifestyle.

If you have been active most days of the week for more than a year, you can start at that level and keep up with the same regimen.

The optimal plan for you fits your lifestyle and allows you to plug yourself in to a realistic and enjoyable program. After all, there is nothing fun about going straight from no activity to running 5 days a week. It is not gradual, it is not fun, and your body will fight you every step of the way.

Take the time to review your activity patterns in your life. Be honest and open. There is no right or wrong answer, only an answer that will start you on the right path—a path that will lead you to greater things.

What is your training goal?

Jane B. Fit: I would like to finish the race in a particular time goal. My sister finished the marathon in 4 hours, and I would like to run with her in the race.

All too often we set our goals based on what we see around us rather than what we have to work with. I have heard this many times. Never having run before, Jane is already setting herself up for failure by (1) wanting to run a marathon and (2) wanting to finish in a specific time.

I am by no means saying she can't run the marathon in 4 hours, but if that is her initial goal, she will fail. Her body is not ready to jump into a marathon. If Jane starts a marathon training program today, she will end up injured and frustrated—a familiar pattern for her.

When selecting a program, be aware if you are type A or ambitious by nature. These characteristics may have motivated you to buy this book, but you'll need to tame your dragons and embark on a more conservative plan that your type A brain will feel comfortable sticking with.

If this is your first long-distance race, enjoy it! Set your goal to finish and take the time to enjoy every step. You will have plenty of time to improve and train for a time goal later.

The training is new, the distance is new, and at some point in the race, every step you take will be new.

If you've completed the distance already, you know you can go the distance and have a better idea of where you are. For you, a specific time goal makes sense. Just keep your rate of improvement gradual. If you ran a 2-hour half-marathon and want to improve your time, set a goal to shed 5 to 10 minutes rather than an entire half-hour. Aim to progress gradually and you will attain your goals.

How many days per week and how much time can you commit to training?

Jane B. Fit: I can commit to training 3–4 days per week and 4–6 hours per week.

Commitment is key while training for long-distance races. You won't need to quit your job and sell your kids to train, but you will need to set aside time on a frequent basis. You may need to re-arrange your daily activities and schedule. You may need to sit down with your family and explain you will need "you time" to achieve your goals. You may even need to tell your coworkers why you are leaving at 5 on the dot.

At the minimum, you must commit 3 to 4 hours per week to train for a half-marathon and 4 to 6 hours per week for a full marathon. It may seem a little daunting now, but after a few weeks, your lifestyle will take a new direction and you will wonder what you used to do with your time during your pre-training days.

Set aside at least one nonworking *day* a week for your longest workout, as well as a half-hour to an hour each of four to five work-days for shorter sessions. That's right. We said an entire day for your longest workout. Though your longest run ever may last only 3 hours, you'll spend the rest of the day preparing nutritionally and mentally for the run and recovering physically, nutritionally, and mentally after the run.

Pick a low-key day—usually on the weekend—that's less stressful to fit in your longest training session. Typically long-distance athletes get the shorter workouts in during the work-week and save the long workout for the weekend, and we designed our training plans around that lifestyle. That said, you have a lot of flexibility in your training program. You can move workouts and rest days to match your schedule. It is all a matter of working with the training principles of progression. We'll ex-plain those later. For now, find the time and put it in your schedule.

What are the top three factors that motivate you to exercise?

Jane B. Fit: I am motivated by working out with friends, following a structured program, and achieving a goal.

Identifying what motivates you will help keep the fires burning during your training program. Jane enjoys training with people and having a goal and program to reach for. She is a good candidate for a local group-training program. She could join Team in Training or any other organized long-distance training group. She can also organize her own intimate group of friends and set off for the trails.

Try to include your motivations in your training in a realistic manner. For example, Jane should train with buddies who have similar goals and are willing to train at her pace. You may be motivated by the time alone or the fitness benefits. List your motivations at the top of your training program and read them often. These are the benefits from your efforts that will keep you moving forward.

What will be your top three challenges to finishing this training program?

Jane B. Fit: I am stretched for time and have a 3-year-old child to care for. Finding the time will be my greatest challenge.

Jane shares a common challenge when committing to train for a long-distance training program. Identifying things that may get in your way will help you to avoid what we call the pitfalls of training. If time is scarce, find a program that fits the time you can carve out. If you struggle to find people to support you in your efforts to achieve goals, surround yourself with a new crowd of people with similar goals. They are out there. All you need to do is find them and make the adjustments.

Know Before You Go

Before you move on to chapter 5, look over your answers in your personal training inventory. Consider how those answers will affect the optimal training program for you. Also, check each answer for honesty. Once you've done that, we can get on with the training. See you soon.

Remember:

- Choosing the right program will allow you to progress faster.
- Choosing the wrong program will result in injury and frustration.
- It's better to do a little too little than a little too much.
- No training plan will keep you dry in the rain.
- Your body responds to the miles you train, not the miles you log.
- Getting support is important, but not essential.
- A little dishonesty today will become a lot of disappointment tomorrow.
- Knowing your limits is more valuable than exceeding them.
- The body you've got is the only body you'll get.
- Age and wisdom are as important as youth and vigor.

Part Two

Training

Choosing the right program

for your body, background,

and goals

CHAPTER FIVE

Anatomy of a Long-Distance Training Program, Part 1

Your long-distance training program includes five important components. How much you focus on each component depends on your needs, genetics, and priorities.

Mortal Dilemma: *Okay, I'm hooked. I've decided to participate in a half- or full marathon. Now what?*

We get e-mail all the time from folks who want to participate in half-marathons or marathons. Too often they write something like, "I just started running 5 weeks ago, and I want to do a marathon this fall. What do you recommend?" When we're not feeling very generous, we write back and recommend first to find a good orthopedic doctor and physical therapist.

You can't just jump into a long-distance training program—

even a modest one like our level one *Marathoning for Mortals* plan—until you give your body a chance to make the adaptations it needs to stay healthy and strong as you keep increasing the training volume and stress. You've got to be willing to spend the months preparing both physically and mentally for the task at hand.

We suggest that you run or walk on a regular basis—and by that we mean getting out and moving at least 30 minutes, three times a week—for at least a year before embarking on any long-distance training program. During that year, you'll build your foundation. After that, you'll strengthen your foundation with up to 6 more months of training before tackling a half- or full marathon.

In other words, if today marked your very first run, you can plan on running a half- or full marathon 1 year and 6 months from today.

Why so long? To keep you from getting injured. We know; we know. You've got a friend who started running in March and completed her first marathon in a Boston qualifying time in May. It happens, but it doesn't happen often. And while it *might* happen for you, we don't think it's worth the risk.

John's Cautionary Tale

I started my first marathon about a year after I started running. I say "started" because it was nearly a full year later before I *finished* my first marathon. So I'm giving you this advice not only as someone who has worked with thousands of new long-distance athletes but also as someone who made just about every possible mistake when I prepared for my first marathon.

First of all, I didn't bother to buy a book about training for long distances. So if you're reading this, you are already way smarter than

I was (unless you're still standing in the bookstore). I was foolish enough to believe that I could construct a training program based on no knowledge of what it would take to run 26.2 miles. After all, I was nearly 45 years old. Surely no one could know more than me.

I did a little calculating. I had seen some formulas in a cycling magazine that suggested—if needed—I could ride three times as far as my normal daily ride or one-third of my average weekly distance. Since there was no way I was going to be running 75 miles a week, I decided to take the former approach. I immediately started running close to 9 miles every time I ran—three times farther than I had ever run before.

Are you with me so far?

Not satisfied with just that approach, I decided that I had to learn to run on tired legs. I didn't know much about marathoning, but I had heard that your legs are really tired at the end. I figured I'd learn how to do that.

My solution? I decided to ride my bicycle for at least 2 hours before I started my long runs. You read that correctly. I rode for 2 hours to fatigue my legs before I started my long runs. Can you see what's coming?

What you've got now is a 45-year-old man who, until this point, had been running for a half-hour at a time for less than a year. This 45-year-old man is now suddenly running for more than 90 minutes at least three times a week. On the weekends, he's biking to near exhaustion and then doing a 3-plus-hour run.

I was so overtrained that even my hair hurt.

As I dragged myself up and down stairs with knees the size of cantaloupes, I actually thought I was doing all the right things. I was training. I was injured. I was in pain. Hey, that's what running long distance is all about. . . . right?

Wrong!

One last little bit of genius: I knew that athletes tapered their mileage before big events, so I decided to try it. I didn't take one running step for an entire week before the marathon. Nothing. *Nada. Niente.* I just sat. I sat and listened to the sound of my entire body locking up.

On race morning, though, I was still deliciously unaware of what was ahead of me. It was a cold, rainy morning with a temperature around freezing. Of course, since I was so well-prepared (I thought) and was going to run so fast and so far (I thought), I wore just a long-sleeved shirt and shorts. Sure, I was cold at the start, but I knew I'd be burning up the course later on.

As so often happens in my life, my stupidity caught up with me when I least expected it. My complete and total ignorance became blindingly clear when, before mile marker 1, my left knee locked up. I don't mean that it got tight. It locked up!

Mortal Miracle

"Motivated to fight middle age and reclaim my love of sport, I joined a training program 2 years ago. I met friends and trained for a half-marathon. And I did it. My goal was to cross the finish line, and I did.

"This year I'm training for a full marathon. I would have told you 'You're crazy!' if you had suggested 2 years ago that I could accomplish all this. But the running helps. My mind is sharper and my friends are more positive. So, you see, I have a secret weapon, and that is the unstoppable enthusiasm of being a runner."

—Jacquie, no age given

There I was, less than 1 mile into it, limping next to the cop on the motorcycle, wondering what in the world I was going to do. I wasn't scheduled to see my support crew until about mile 6. The answer was as obvious as it was painful. I was going to have to move to the sidewalk and limp for the next hour and a half. And that's exactly what I did. I made it to mile 7 before I could no longer limp. Then I got in the car and went home.

What did I do wrong? Coach Jenny will soon take a shot at answering that question, but looking back with 33 marathons under my belt, I can spot a few mistakes.

First, I didn't respect the distance, and second, I didn't listen to my body. Let's look at these separately.

Respecting the distance. The training volume needed to successfully complete a half- or full marathon is enough to injure anyone's body. It's a lot of time on your feet, over your knees and hips, and swinging your arms. The total distance recommended in many of the training programs approaches 700 miles over the span of 4, 5, or even 6 months. That's nearly the distance from Chicago to Washington, D.C. It's a l-o-n-g way.

I didn't respect the distance enough to let it slowly become a part of my daily life. I just made the mental switch to marathon training and dragged my body along with me. It didn't work.

Listening to my body. I'm not going to try to kid anyone about this. I was injured. I was hurting. I knew it. I was taking medication to help me stand the pain and keep running. I was putting chemicals inside my body, outside my body, and everywhere around my body.

I knew. I knew from the first whisper of pain from my knee that I was pushing myself too far, too fast. I knew from the first telltale ache that wouldn't go away no matter how much anti-inflammatory medication I took. I knew.

You'll know, too.

Progress Without Pain

I think many of us believe, as John did for much of his early running career, that we must feel pain in order to achieve.

I've heard similar stories from many athletes. Once, a woman joined my program who wanted desperately to run without injury. When we began examining her personal inventory, I quickly realized what we were up against. She was running away from her problems and letting her emotions rule her training.

She had a plan, and she stuck right to it. Her problem wasn't motivation; her problem was being so out of touch with her body

---

Mortal Miracle

"The thought of running a half-marathon, 13.1 miles, always seemed impossible. I had a hard time running 1 mile, let alone 13.1! When I learned that I could alternate running and walking, all the negatives instantly became positives. I felt my spirits, enthusiasm, and determination lift. Finally, I was learning a tool to head me toward an achievement that only ever seemed like a dream.

"As we trained, I learned the run/walk technique, and each week, each mile became easier and easier. The excitement was hard to contain, especially when we passed runners at mile 7, 8, 9 during training. For the first time I could say to myself, 'I'm going to do this.' The haunting negative 'No' voice in my head had disappeared.

"Now I stand tall and confident; my head and heart are ringing with a continuous, positive 'Yes,' a joy that everyone should have the opportunity to feel."

—Tina, age 33

that she ran right through knee pain, back pain, and eventually hip pain. Her primary pains developed secondary pains, and soon she was moving so slowly that she could barely run. It was almost as if she felt she deserved to feel the pain.

And she was a seasoned runner! I share this with you to let you in to the minds and bodies of seasoned runners. They are not all right, they are not all doing the correct training, and some are even using the training to escape the more daunting aspects of their lives. Don't emulate these runners!

Think of your long-distance training program as a blueprint for a home you are building. You'll start with a blueprint—drawn up by us—that includes the long run/walk, the shorter workouts, the rest days, the cross-training, and so on. It is all there in front of you from the beginning. But once the program begins, so does the shuffling. Training days may shift, for example, or aches and pains may delay a long workout for a week.

Just as in building a home, you will encounter factors that you can and cannot control along the way. So start with a blueprint, but let the training unfold naturally with all the peaks and valleys. Just as you would never push a project to the point where the quality suffers, you should not push your training to the point of burnout or injury. You can't play catch-up in long-distance training, but you can modify days, workouts, and mileage.

Your blueprint for a long-distance training program includes the following five important rooms.

1. The living room. We call this room *the long, slow workout.* Like the living room in your house, you will spend much of your time on this workout. The long workout starts with low miles and continues to build gradually throughout the duration of the program. This workout helps you develop endurance and teaches your body to use fat as a primary and limitless source of energy.

The long, slow workout prepares the body, mind, and spirit for the big day. Every week you will go a little farther, and every workout will prepare your body to stay vertical for hours on end. We're talking 3 or more hours on end. I call this "foot time."

2. The bathroom. Bathrooms allow us to multitask. You can get ready for the day, shower, shave, prepare to go to bed, and—well—"clean out the plumbing," if you will. The multitasking room in your training plan includes your *shorter workouts* done, typically, during the week. For some training programs, these shorter workouts may include a balanced mix of faster and slower workouts. For other programs, these workouts will serve as memory sessions, sessions that remind the body—muscles, bones, and cardiovascular system—how to run or walk. The bathroom is centrally located in your home and the short workouts connect the long workouts together each week.

3. The recreation room. Just as the rec room allows you to turn off the overworked areas of your brain while you use other areas of your brain to play a variety of games, *active rest days and cross-training* allow your run and walk muscles to go on a minivacation but still remain involved.

Cross-training includes any activity other than walking or running. Your distance muscles become secondary "helpers" while cycling, swimming, strength training, performing yoga postures, or even inline skating. Spending time in the rec room allows your mind to focus on something other than right-left-right-left and provides a well-earned rest for your distance muscles. More important, active rest helps balance your body along the way. If you've ever pulled weeds for a day, you understand what I mean. Repeating the same sequence over and over completely fatigues one set of muscles. You wake the next day unable to move without whimpering. You'll learn more about cross-training in chapter 10.

4. The bedroom. This includes your ***rest days and weeks***. Rest is something that you will need to do early and often. It will roll evenly throughout your training. Remember that it during the downtime that your body adapts and grows stronger. I mention this because once you get going on your training regimen, believe it or not, you just may have a hard time resting.

When you see "rest" on your training program, it doesn't mean staying up late and reading in bed or getting in a short run just for insurance. Rest means rest. It means going to bed, turning off the lights, and catching some z's. Most of all, it means *no* running.

Rest weeks will be subtler. Rest weeks include a normal training pattern but with fewer miles. I call these "cutback weeks." A reduction in overall weekly mileage allows your body to adapt to the stress of the increases. It is a little like climbing a mountain. You will spend time climbing in elevation, and then you will traverse along a ridge for a while. You are still moving, but just not up!

5. The kitchen. Here you'll find the ***nutritional*** component of your training. You are what you eat. Some of you may spend lots of time in the kitchen while others spend not nearly enough. The act of eating can be locked up in emotional nurturing for one athlete and starvation for another. Regardless of whether or not you have a healthy relationship with food, this program will teach you to view food as fuel and eating as a necessary part of training.

Nutrition is the fuel that keeps your program running. You won't go anywhere or run very well without good nutrition.

A Reflection of You

Your training program, much like your house, will ultimately be a reflection of you. While there are certain aspects of the training program that must be there, make sure to put some of your favorite "things" around your training house. If, for example, you've had a weekly habit of eating ice cream with the family every Friday evening, don't eliminate that just because you're in a training program. The key to being able to live in your new training house will be making it comfortable.

You now can read the blueprint to the rooms in your training program. You're ready to look at the electrical wiring, the hidden parts in each room that play a vital role in the training process.

Know Before You Go

In chapter 6, you'll learn more details about the right elements of a training program. Before you move on, however, promise yourself that you will dedicate the same amount of time and effort to each room in your training house. Rather than spending all of your time in the living room racking up long run miles, promise to also spend your nights in the bedroom and some days in the rec room.

Remember:

- A long-distance training program starts with a solid foundation.
- You should be active for a year before starting a long-distance training program.
- How long it took someone else to train doesn't mean anything to you.
- Pain is *not* a part of a long-distance training program.
- Respect the distance.
- Listen to your body, even if you don't like what it's telling you.
- Training is a journey, not an escape.
- If the plan isn't working, change the plan.
- The long workout is the cornerstone of your training.
- Improvement comes during your rest days.

CHAPTER SIX

Anatomy of a Long-Distance Training Program, Part 2

It may be true that a journey of 1,000 miles begins with a single step, but the journey to the finish line begins first with a plan and then a single step. Start on the right foot by taking the time to understand the elements of your training program.

Mortal Dilemma: *I've looked at other training programs. They all seem so complicated. How can I train if I can't even figure out what the workouts are?*

—⚏—

In the last chapter, we explained the basic elements in your training program. Every week you'll include one longer workout, some shorter workouts, some cross-training, some rest, and good nutrition.

But how does that all fit together? Exactly what should you do during each type of workout, and how often should you do it?

We'll now attempt to answer those questions. In chapter 5, we looked at your training landscape from far away, from a satellite's perspective. Now let's zoom in a little closer to sharpen your view.

Workouts are a lot like restaurant menus. Just as there are various cuisines, there are stages of a workout. Following a training program can be as complex as trying to read a foreign menu or as easy as ordering the special of the day.

Appetizer: Warmup

Every workout, long or short, begins with a warmup. Like an appetizer before your main course, the warmup prepares your body for your main workout.

Just as an appetizer before a main course gets your digestive juices flowing, your warmup before your main workout gets your blood flowing. It gradually increases your breathing rate, heart rate, and blood flow to your working muscles. Starting too fast will produce breathlessness, premature fatigue, muscle pulls, side stitches, and possibly an injury that could sideline your marathon training.

Your warmup for all of your marathon running and walking workouts—long or short—will be the same. You'll start with an easy walk. You'll walk comfortably for 5 minutes. During this time as your body directs blood flow to your muscles, you'll *feel* yourself warm up. Your body will generate heat.

This is especially important when training in the morning, as your muscles are cold and shortened from sleeping all night. Your body will perform much more efficiently if you progress gradually from first gear to second and then third.

Main Course: Meat of the Workout

The main course of your training program is the time you spend walking or running for a specific duration, time, and intensity. Every workout has a specific purpose. Every workout is unique and provides just one piece of the long-distance training puzzle.

The endurance workout, otherwise known as the "long" one (remember: the living room of your house) provides the "meat and potatoes" of the program. The main course of this workout will take quite a long time to complete.

Mortal Miracle

"It took me 3 hours, 2 minutes, and 38 seconds to run/race walk a half-marathon. Less than a year before, I would have said that I could never do such a thing. I, the fat girl, was actually running—and liking it. I had tried running many years ago without success. At the time I thought athletic women all were skinny with narrow hips and small breasts. I assumed that a woman like me couldn't run.

"As I neared the finish area, I saw a crowd of people lining the street, applauding and shouting. I looked behind me to see whom they were applauding for. There wasn't anybody there! I burst into tears. I just started sobbing. I was overwhelmed by the realization that I had actually done it. I had finished the 13.1-mile half-marathon.

"I finished number 565. There were 40 more behind me! I had met my goal. I had finished."

—Kathryn, age 54

Your long run prepares your body for the mileage on race day. Because each long workout gets—well—longer, you will need to devote progressively more time to complete it as you near marathon race day. That's why we suggest you complete your long run on a day off, when work responsibilities won't interfere with your workout responsibilities.

Though you'll increase the main course of your long workout in distance and time each week, you'll do so gradually. This gradual progression allows your body to seamlessly adapt to the increase in mileage.

The long workout increases in small increments week to week, with the longest session 3 weeks prior to the race. The workout increases your cardiovascular endurance, which is the ability of your body to use oxygen efficiently over time; mentally prepares you to go the distance; and prepares your muscles, tendons, and joints for the impact with time on your feet.

In our programs, you'll never increase your long workout time more than 10 percent per week. In other words, if you are active for 60 minutes this week, next week you can add *only* 6 minutes to your long workout time. It sounds painfully slow, but the 10 percent rule will help you avoid pain of overworked muscles, tendons, and joints.

In our walk/run and run/walk programs, you will mix and match the running motion and the walking motion during the main course of each session, whether you're going long or short. Both are important and the goal is to find a mix of walking and running or running and walking that works best for you. We will make some recommendations in the programs, but view these as guidelines only, not absolutes.

—ᴍ—

For me, John, running for 5 minutes and walking for 1 minute creates the perfect mix for long-distance events. I've used this mix in more than 15 marathons and many half-marathons. I've been able to finish in my time goal (when I had one) and still feel great, ready to run and walk again in just a few days.

At first glance, you may look at the tail end of the program and think to yourself, "Self, how in the heck am I going to complete 10 or 20 miles?" No worries. Training for a long-distance race is cyclical, with peaks and valleys. In general, the long workouts build for a few weeks and then decrease to allow you to rest and recover. The long workout is the most important, but it can also be the most daunting. Progress 1 day at a time, 1 week at a time and soon you will be saying, "I have to do only an 8-miler this weekend."

Steamed Vegetables: Cutback Weeks

We've woven rest weeks throughout all of the training programs. These weeks arc a lot like vegetables. They do you a lot of good, even if it doesn't secm that way.

Every few weeks on your training program, you'll lower your overall mileage. After a few weeks of building miles, you'll probably welcome these lower-mileage weeks with open arms. In fact, your cutback week will probably feel like a vacation when compared to the week of hard training that came before.

Use these cutback weeks wisely and follow the mileage prescribed. Though many of you will savor these lower-mileage weeks, we know that some of you will feel tempted to skip them. Training too hard or longer than prescribed will lead only to disaster. Your body, brain, career, and relationships all benefit from cutback weeks. Use these periodic lower-mileage weeks to catch up with family, spend more time at the office, or even go to the movies. Just don't use them to add more miles to your training!

In addition to cutback weeks, we've also included rest days in each schedule. A rest day means moving about your normal day without any structured exercise. Rest does not mean lying on a couch all day while eating bonbons. Just as you must sleep at night to rejuvenate

---

The Three Constants

Each of our training programs contains elements that are fundamental to all long-distance training. They include:

The 10 percent rule. In every program, at every level, you add no more than 10 percent to your total time or distance from one week to the next.

A workout sequence. For every program, the "rule of sequence" is the same. That means you must adhere to the sequence of the workouts even if you miss one (or two). If you have to miss a speed workout, for example, you just miss it and go on; don't try to make it up later. The same is true with your long workouts. You may miss one weekend. If you do, you just skip it and go on. Don't try to sneak it in sometime in the middle of the next week.

A taper. Just as the programs all build mileage gradually, the final stages of all the programs and one of the most important pieces of the training puzzle is the taper. The taper is when you start backing off your mileage and intensity in preparation for the big day. For most programs, this will be the last 3 weeks. Those 3 weeks are emotionally difficult even if they are physically easy. But don't worry: In coming chapters, we're going to give you some tips on how to survive the taper period.

your body for tomorrow, you must occasionally take a break from your training. Rest days rejuvenate your body for your next workout.

In our training programs, your rest days will follow longer or more intense workouts. They'll allow your tattered muscles to repair any nicks or dents you may have inflicted during your long run. They'll allow your brain to take a break from its tireless job of motivating your body to move. They'll allow your entire body to grow stronger. Rest allows your body to recover from the stress and impact of the training cycle. Your body can't go too long without adequate sleep and can't train optimally without rest days.

Rest days are deceiving. At first you may think, "Great! I get to rest all these days. What a treat." Yet once you've committed yourself fully to your training program, you'll strangely find it harder and harder to take a break. It's almost as if you'll be in a rhythm and won't want to stop. Too many runners and walkers skip their rest days and ultimately end up watching the race from the sidelines because of injury. Your rest days are just as important as all your other workouts.

Fresh Ground Pepper: Cross-Training

Like pepper, cross-training adds flavor to your training program.

We often refer to cross-training as active rest because it allows your long-distance muscles a little nap time while activating the often neglected opposing muscles. Cross-training for long-distance training includes any movement other than walking and running. You can cycle, swim, strength train, row, practice yoga, take group exercise classes, inline skate. . . . this list goes on and on.

You have many options. Select an activity that you enjoy, as cross-training should give you a mental and physical time-out from the structure and intensity of your long-distance program. Consider it a mini–training vacation.

We've strategically placed cross-training throughout all of the training programs to balance your "moving muscles" to avoid overuse injuries. Cross-training exercises your non-long-distance muscles and aids in muscular balance. For this reason, we refer to cross-training as active rest days. You are able to rest your training muscles while stimulating the cardiovascular system and using less used muscles.

You'll learn more about cross-training in chapter 10.

Hot Sauce: Tempo Workouts

We've scattered faster workouts throughout the marathon training programs in the form of something called tempo workouts. Like hot sauce, these will really spice up your training.

The tempo workout will improve your speed, efficiency, and form. There are three tempo workouts called A, B, and C. You'll learn more about the specifics of each workout as we get into the training programs. What's important about all tempo workouts is that they will teach your body and your brain to relax as you get into the upper effort limits.

You run all of your tempo workouts just below your anaerobic threshold, that is, the level at which your body begins to burn the short supply of glycogen or sugar in your system at a higher rate. Your muscles can burn one of two types of fuel—fat or glycogen (stored carbohydrates). At lower intensities—such as walking—your muscles prefer to burn mostly fat for fuel. However, the higher your intensity, the more glycogen your muscles burn.

You can go for days on fat stores but only a few hours on glycogen. The body is always using a ratio of both, but for the purpose of a successful and comfortable race, you want to burn at a higher rate of fat.

Your tempo workouts will allow you to raise your threshold. Ultimately, your body will burn a higher percentage of fat for a longer period of time at a higher intensity. This not only helps you lose weight; it also bolsters your endurance. The more your body burns fat for fuel, the more it conserves glycogen and the longer you can run without feeling tired.

Table Manners: Form Drills

You don't want to look like a country bumpkin at a fancy dinner, do you? Specific sessions that focus on your running posture and form—whether walking or running—will help you to run your "nonform" workouts with a better cadence, posture, and footstrike. As a result, you'll make a huge impact on your race time, performance, fatigue level, and risk of injury. Maintaining strong form throughout training and racing will allow you to move faster and farther with less energy expenditure.

Picture a sleek, aerodynamic car whisking down an expressway with very little resistance. Now picture the same car with a huge luggage rack on top, the windows open, and a child hanging a wind sock out the window. Both cars are moving at the same speed, but one is using more energy to get from one place to the next.

Your form is the same. The next time you work out, take a look at other walkers and runners around you. What are the stronger people doing with their arms, legs, and torsos? How does that differ from the slower people?

Proper form can save you precious energy and time. That is why we've dedicated an entire workout to form.

Form provides your secret formula for quick improvement. Most beginning long-distance athletes don't think about proper form and head out the door to run as fast and as far as possible. If you begin with developing the basics, you will pass them on race day and feel much stronger in the process.

As our good friend and fellow coach Brendan Cournane repeats every season, "Your form will carry you through." The first parts of your body that tend to lose proper form during the long run are your torso and stride length. If you don't believe this, watch the end of a marathon. You'll see lots of people bent over and dragging their feet inch by inch. You now know the secret, and you have the knowledge to move efficiently and optimize your time and efforts. More important, you will look good for the finish line photos.

One type of form drills, called strides, captures this type of carefree movement. These short drills will help improve your running and walking mechanics. They don't consume a lot of time but will require genuine effort and focus.

After completing your walking cooldown, perform four strides with 1 minute of easy walking in between to catch your breath. Gradually increase your speed for 20 to 30 seconds, focusing on quick foot turnover and extending your stride length. You should feel as if you are completing the shuttle run or 100-yard dash in the schoolyard. Gradually increase your pace and then gradually decrease your pace. Strides are not all-out sprints but rather controlled fast walking and running. Strides for the walkers and walk/runners should include walking. Run/walkers and runners perform the strides with running.

While striding, think about your form. Increase your stride length and reach your feet farther on each step, but maintain the quick footstrike frequency. This is how you get stronger. This is how you get faster—one stride at a time. There is a proper way to walk and run. You need to learn the basics before you sign up for the big show.

Side Dishes: Shorter Workouts

In addition to your longer runs, tempo sessions, cross-training, and form drills, you'll also complete a few workouts each week that will add to your total weekly mileage.

These shorter running and walking workouts during the week are maintenance and recovery sessions. We often call them muscle memory sessions because they remind the body and mind how to run and walk. The shorter workouts also aid in recovery from the long workouts by improving blood flow and circulation to the training muscles. The shorter workouts bridge the gap between the long workouts week to week.

Like side dishes, these will change in length and intensity from week to week. Use them to keep your workouts fresh and interesting. No one wants to eat cole slaw with every meal.

Wine: Workout Intensity

Just as too strong a wine overcomes or detracts from the taste of your food, a workout that is too intense can overcome all of your training benefits.

For every workout in our training programs, we suggest you complete it at a specific intensity. You can monitor your intensity in one of three ways.

1. Mentally deciding whether you're moving at a conversational, moderate, or hard pace
2. Monitoring your heart rate
3. Using something called the I-Rate scale

You can pick whichever of the three methods works best for you. To understand how each works, let's take a look at the right intensity of a long, slow workout.

The intensity of the long workout should be comfortably slow. This is critical to monitor your pace and keep it consistent. That's a conversational pace. You should be able to recount detailed stories of your grade-school teachers to your running buddy—without feeling winded.

If you are using a heart rate monitor, keep your rate between 60 and 75 percent of your estimated maximum heart rate. In other words, go at a pace at which you can have a conversation but not sing a song. (You'll find out how to use a heart rate monitor and how to calculate your maximum heart rate in chapter 7.)

Another way to monitor your pace is to use the I-Rate system. Rate how you feel on a scale from 1 to 10, with 1 equaling complete rest and 10 equaling an all-out effort.

For your long workout, keep your intensity at an I-Rating of 6 to 7.5. Any higher and you will pay a price. I've witnessed too many runners training at race pace every week. They come out to train and end up racing. This eventually takes a toll on the body over time. It breaks down and is not able to recover. Burnout, fatigue, and slower times are the outcome of training too fast during the long workout.

For all of the workouts listed in our training plans, we suggest a specific intensity. Here's the basic rule of thumb for each.

Shorter workouts. In order for the shorter workouts to benefit your training, complete them at an easy pace, at 6 to 7.5 on the I-Rate scale, or at 60 to 75 percent of your maximum heart rate.

Cross-training. Complete cross-training workouts at an I-Rate of 6 or 7 or at a heart rate of 60 to 70 percent of your maximum. Remember that this is active rest. Completing the workout at anything more than a moderate pace will defeat the purpose of the restful activity. Enjoy it; don't race it.

Tempo sessions. Do your tempo speed workouts at an I-Rate of 8 or at a heart rate of 80 percent of your maximum. The danger here is in pushing too hard for too long. Tempo pace is just outside your comfort zone, comfortably hard. You should be able to talk in short, choppy sentences—"See Jane run" or "Yes" and "No." If you can't speak, slow down. The secret to this workout is to maintain a pace at the threshold. Going beyond it defeats the purpose. If all goes well, your tempo pace will increase over time. Like a report card, this is how you know if you are progressing or regressing.

Dessert: Cooldown

You conclude every good meal with dessert. As my mother says, "It takes the taste away." The cooldown is the dessert of your training. Every workout, long or short, should end with a gradual slowing of pace and intensity. It is the reverse of the warmup.

Slowing down for 5 minutes allows your body to come back to reality, decreasing your breathing and heart rate and bringing blood circulation to its resting point. Take 5 minutes, slow your pace, and relish in your short-term achievements. This will not only aid in quick recovery, but also bring you back to earth with a smile on your face.

Once you're back to reality, take a few more minutes to stretch your fatigued muscles. This is the best time to stretch because your muscles are warm and therefore more pliable. An analogy I like to use involves a piece of chewing gum. If you chew the gum, take it out, and stretch it, the gum will extend without snapping. It is warm and stretches easily. If you take that same piece of gum out of your mouth, place it on a desk, and come back 10 minutes later to stretch it, the gum will snap almost immediately. It is cold, less pliable, and unyielding. Muscles work the same way.

Save the stretching for the end of the cooldown, when your workout is complete and your muscles are still warm. Include stretches for your moving muscles in your upper body, chest, back, and shoulders as well as core muscles in the low back, abdomen, and the muscles that will put up the most resistance: the hamstrings, quadriceps, and calves.

Maintaining and improving flexibility will have a direct effect on your recovery. Flexibility also has a positive or negative effect on your stride length. Tight hamstrings and calf muscles shorten the length of your stride. Mile after mile, your body has to work harder to get where it is going. Take the time to stretch, and you will extend your performance and enhance your quality of life.

Know Before You Go

Now you know *almost* everything you need to take your first step into the world of the long-distance athlete. In chapter 7, you'll discover the final piece of the training puzzle to help you monitor your intensity during your workouts. In chapter 8, you'll pick your training program. Then you'll take your first step.

Remember:

- Training programs are only as complicated as you make them.
- Choose a training program that suits your taste.
- Each element of the training program has a purpose.
- The training effect occurs while you rest.
- The long workout is the foundation of a long-distance training program.
- Cross-training allows your muscles to get stronger without injury.
- Speed work improves your efficiency.
- When all else fails, your form will carry you through.
- The right intensity will yield the right results.
- You can skip a workout, but don't change the sequence.

CHAPTER SEVEN

You Gotta Have Heart

Going faster is just a matter of trying harder, right?

Nope. It might have been true in the fifth grade, but as an adult, you need to learn to train smarter, not harder.

Mortal Dilemma: *I see people wearing heart rate monitor straps around their chests. Isn't that kind of training only for the fast runners?*

A few years ago I, John, was working with one of the major manufacturers of heart rate monitors. The project, which was a lot of fun, was that I would allow them to "monitor" my heart rate while I ran a marathon.

The morning after the event, I called to find out why my results weren't posted on their Web site. They told me that the experiment was a total failure. Something must have been wrong with my transmitter, they told me. All of the data were wrong.

When I asked what was wrong, they said, "Well, from the data, it looks as if you started off at about 65 percent of your maximum heart rate—which we would expect—but then you pushed it up and it looks like your effort was at about 80 percent of your max for nearly 5 hours."

"That's right," I said. "That's the way I run marathons." Their response has become my mantra. "Do you know how fit you'd have to be to keep your heart rate at 80 percent for nearly 5 hours?" they asked in disbelief.

"I *am* fit!" I yelled. "I'm just slow."

The truth is that—despite popular belief—those of us who get out there and spend 4, 5, 6, or more hours running and walking marathons are very fit. We're just slow.

Many people—and perhaps you are one of them—erroneously think that a runner's pace correlates directly with that same runner's effort level. Those who worked at the heart rate monitor company believed this. They thought that the reason I was so slow was because I really wasn't trying very hard. They're wrong. I do try hard. For me, with my history and genetics, a 5-hour marathon is a very hard effort.

It turns out that the effort put forth by all long-distance athletes is about the same. What's different is their speed. Effort is the constant. Pace is the variable.

It's not nearly as complicated as it sounds. You've got a heart; you might as well know how it works and how to make it work better for you.

The Elements of Effort and Intensity

Sometimes the language used to describe the elements of effort can be confusing. Let's take a minute and run down some of the most common concepts and try to make sense out of them.

Maximum heart rate. This is—steady now—your *maximum* heart rate. (I told you this stuff wasn't hard.) Your maximum is the fastest your heart will beat under any circumstances. Your max isn't related to what you're doing. Your max will be the same whether you're running, biking, or falling out of an airplane.

Your max is at its highest the day you're born. For most male babies, it's about 220 beats per minute. For female babies, it's closer to 226. Year by year over the course of your lifetime, your max heart rate goes down. And there's not much you can do about it.

The old formulas, the ones where you subtract your age from 220, don't work well. That formula assumes that you are losing one heart beat per year off your max. It turns out that chronically fit people lose closer to one beat every 2 years.

Determining your honest-to-goodness maximum heart rate involves a very strenuous test. You've got to be willing and able to place enough demand on your heart to get it to beat as fast as it can. I've done it. It wasn't pretty.

In fact, I had the test done on a treadmill and a stationary bike about a week apart. At the time, I wasn't convinced that my max was my max. I was sure that my running max would be different than my biking max. Guess what? I was wrong. They were identical.

The safest way to identify your own personal maximum heart rate is to ask your doctor to schedule a maximum stress test. Most sports medicine facilities can also provide a physician-monitored test as well. Depending on the lab, they may even hook you up and monitor your air expired to calculate fun things like oxygen processed, aerobic threshold, and CO_2 expired.

The easiest way to find out your maximum heart rate is to purchase a heart rate monitor and hit the roads. Sign up for a local 5-K, strap on your shoes and heart rate monitor, and conduct your own science experiment.

Warm up prior to the race with a few easy and slow minutes, take the first mile at a moderate pace and the second at a challenging pace, and finish the last 1.1 miles at a pace you can't wait to stop.

Watch your monitor and keep track of the highest number throughout the entire race. This will be your maximum heart rate.

Sure, it's not as accurate as the doctor's lab, but it's a lot more valid than plugging in your age to a formula.

You'll find more information on what to look for when purchasing a monitor in chapter 12.

Resting heart rate. This is—you guessed it—your *resting* heart rate. (Wondering why you were ever worried about this stuff?) This

---

The Mortal Runner's Heart

I (*Jenny*) always get a smile on my face when I hear the chatter. It is usually at a family function, where I stand out like an alien from Mars. They say, "There she is, that runner girl." They tell themselves that running is bad for you to make themselves feel better about their lack of activity. "All that running is going to hurt her organs," they say. "Heck, Vern, I've even heard that when a woman runs, her uterus will drop over time."

Oh boy, I've heard them all, but my absolute favorite family picnic comment story is "I don't exercise because I know I have a limited number of beats in my life and I don't want them to run out." That is classic. Then they go into a dissertation about Jim Fixx having a heart attack because he was a runner. I used to defend my position for the good of the sport, but now I let them have their voice because I know it is more about their fears and less about my running.

The fact is that Jim Fixx lived a very healthy life and had a tremendously deep family history of heart disease. His running prolonged his life, but he couldn't completely outrun his genetics. He died of a heart attack sooner than most, but later than most in his own family.

The facts are simple. The fitter your heart and the stronger your heart, the more efficient your heart.

used to be called your morning heart rate until they figured out that some of you "morning" people wake up already revved up. Your resting heart rate, also known as your basal heart rate, is the minimum number of beats per minute that your heart has to use just to keep you alive.

It's also the best indicator of your overall fitness. In general, people who are fitter will have lower resting heart rates. The stronger your heart is, the stronger it beats. The stronger your heart beats, the higher the volume of blood your heart pumps per beat. The more blood your heart pumps per beat, the fewer beats your heart must take to do its job. Whatever your resting heart rate is today, chances are, as you get fitter, it will drop.

Your resting heart rate is also the best indicator of whether you have recovered from a hard workout or if you're coming down with an illness. Anytime that number starts to creep up on you, look for the explanation. A higher-than-usual morning or resting heart beat may signal that you need more rest days in your schedule, for example.

Cardiac reserve. Okay, this one's a bit more difficult to explain. Your cardiac reserve is the difference between your maximum heart rate and your resting heart rate. So if your max is 180 beats per minute and your resting heart rate is 80 beats per minute, your cardiac reserve is 100 beats per minute.

What's important about your cardiac reserve is that it represents the amount of your heartbeat that you get to use for training. Since your max is a fixed rate that you can't change, the only way to increase your cardiac reserve is to lower your resting heart rate.

Are you with me so far?

Aerobic zone. Aerobic means "in the presence of oxygen." When your heart is beating below about 80 percent of your max, you are in the aerobic zone. This is *the* zone where all the great fat burning takes place. So it's the zone you want to be in if weight management is important to you. This is also the zone in which you can maintain effort over a longer period of time. Go above it and you'll hit the wall—fast.

Anaerobic zone. This is still simple. The opposite of *aerobic*, *anaerobic*, is "not in the presence of oxygen." For most of us, this is when your heart is beating over 80 percent of its maximum. You know this zone. This is when you start to suck air, when your sentences get short; you find it hard to breath and impossible to talk.

In the anaerobic zone, your body switches from using a higher percentage of fat and begins to burn off precious stores of glycogen, something you can run out of very quickly. You do *not* want to spend very much time in this zone. It might seem like fun for a little while. It's a great way to work up a sweat and get all red in the face, but other than making it easy to complain at the end of your workout, there's not that much good in going anaerobic very often.

Lactic acid. This is the exhaust that your muscles produce when they fire. It's like the exhaust on your car. The muscles work hard and produce a toxic by-product called lactic acid. The harder and faster the muscles work, the more lactic acid they produce. Sprinters build up a high percentage of lactic acid in a short period of time because of their dynamic intensity. In a short time, they are forced to shut down and stop. Long-distance athletes train and race at an intensity that allows the body to filter through and remove most of the lactic acid as it's created.

Anaerobic threshold. This is the point of exertion, or heart rate, at which your body can no longer exhaust the lactic acid out of your muscles. Unlike your car, your body's exhaust pipe isn't big enough to clear out all the lactic acid if your effort level gets too high too quickly.

At about 80 percent of max, the lactic acid starts to pool in the muscles. As your muscles fill, they get harder and harder to move, and before you know it you feel like you're running in a bowl of Jell-O.

Here's the fun thing about your anaerobic threshold: It's not constant. You can improve it with the right training. Improving your anaerobic threshold is what allows you to progress from running 3 miles in 40 minutes while being able to chat to completing the same distance in 30 minutes while holding that same conversation.

Getting F.I.T.T.

That's the basic language of effort-based training. The other piece of the lexicon that will help you is a quick explanation of the "F.I.T.T." principle. It comes down to Frequency, Intensity, Time, and Type. These days, we tend to use duration for time and mode for type, but somehow the "F.I.D.M." principle just doesn't have the same pizzazz.

◆ Frequency: how often
◆ Intensity: how hard of an effort
◆ Duration: how long the effort lasts
◆ Mode: activity or form of exercise

All of these are important, but the most important are intensity and duration. These two are linked, inversely, in a way that can't be separated. The higher the duration, the lower the intensity. The higher the intensity, the lower the duration.

Too often, people make the mistake of trying to do too high an intensity workout for too long a duration. No good can come from pushing your heart rate into the stratosphere for a long time for no reason. If you're being chased by a bear, maybe. But for a long-distance training program, definitely not.

Just as often, however, new athletes make the mistake of not spending enough time at the lower intensity. As you start to construct a long-distance training plan, you'll see that the long, slow workouts are designed to be long and slow. If you don't go slow enough, you won't be able to go long enough, and you won't get the benefits that you're after.

The Training Pyramid

Ready to try to put this into some kind of program? Let's look at the Training Pyramid below.

Phase IV
Racing
Intensity: 95% of max heart rate
Benefits: Few for endurance mortals
Good for mortals who want to burn themselves out

Phase III
Economy
Intensity: 85–95% of max heart rate
Benefits: Better form, more efficient stride
Good for seasoned mortals with a strong mileage base

Phase II
Stamina
Intensity: 75–85% of max heart rate
Benefits: Stronger heart, faster speed, better health
Good for seasoned mortals with a strong mileage base

Phase I
Endurance
Intensity: 60–75% of max heart rate
Benefits: Better aerobic base, stronger legs, less fatigue, better fat burning
Good for all mortals

The lowest end of the pyramid is Phase I (60 to 75 percent of your max heart rate). This is the *endurance* element of any successful training program. Since this is a low-intensity workout, it will have to be a high-duration workout.

These are the training days during which you are working on building your aerobic (with oxygen) base. These are the fat-burning workouts that will help teach your body how to use the thousands of calories of stored fat that we all have.

Here's another way to think of the Phase I workout. These train your legs. All you want to do is repeat the muscle action a few hundred times per mile. You don't want to be putting a strain on any other system, like your heart or lungs. These are low-intensity, low-effort workouts.

When done correctly, these training sessions should leave you feeling relaxed and ready to go. The longer the miles, the slower you have to avoid putting pressure on the rest of your body. In time, it may even feel like you're in autopilot mode.

Next up the pyramid is Phase II or *stamina* (75 to 85 percent of max). Great for your heart, these workouts allow you to run or walk at a higher effort. You feel like you're pushing yourself just a little, and they can be a lot of fun. The truth is that most new athletes do all of their workouts in Phase II.

Think about your daily runs or walks. Do you get out there and start going fast enough to make your heart pound right away? Do you like to hear yourself starting to breathe harder? Do you like the feeling that you're pushing yourself? That's all well and good, except you're probably overtraining.

Moving up the pyramid means that these sessions, because they are at a higher effort level, have to be for a shorter duration. You can't—no one can—maintain that high a level of effort on a regular basis. And you don't want to.

One more step up is Phase III or *economy* (85 to 95 percent of max). These are the track sessions or speed workouts. This is where you learn to be a better runner or walker, where you learn to go faster with the same effort or just as fast with less effort.

These sessions can be a lot of fun if you approach them the right way. Make them very short in duration (maybe once around a track for starters) and at an intensity level that will really get your attention. If you've never done speed work at the track, you owe it to yourself to give it a try.

Finally comes Phase IV or peak performance or *racing* (95 percent of max and above). This is the pain and agony stage that most of us never need to experience. You might. You might discover that you've got an enormous untapped reserve of talent that will catapult you into the prize money at your first race. Maybe. It's more likely that you'll find yourself up in that zone at the end of a shorter distance race when you're determined not to let a 7-year-old beat you!

Mortal Miracle

"Few sports allow first-timers and other amateurs to compete on the very same playing field in the very same event as the elite athletes. Running is one of these sports. Few people can say that they completed the same 26.2 miles as a world-class athlete. But that's just what I did, along with 24,000 of my closest friends at the October 1999 Chicago Marathon. Khalid Khannouchi broke the then-world record in a race in which I was a participant! My life has changed merely knowing that I can compete with, but not against, the elite athletes."

—Gloria, age 43

The Proof Is in the Heart Rate Monitor

Still not convinced that effort-based, time-not-mileage training is the way to go? Okay, let's take a look at some other training methods.

Our favorite is the "hard day-easy day" protocol. You've seen it or at least heard of it. You go out and bust your butt one day, then take an easy day the next day. On the weekends you do a long run at your predicted race pace and add mileage as the program goes on. It sounds good on paper, but there's one small problem.

Define "easy." Define "hard." And don't start in with the "I know it when I feel it" rationale!

John has run 33 marathons. Does that mean that running a marathon is *easy* for him? No! Just as there's no way to judge hard or easy based on distance, there's also no way to judge hard or easy based on pace. Is a 7-minute-per-mile pace easy? Maybe for a world-class marathoner, but not for either of us. Is a 12-minute pace hard? Yes, if your normal daily pace is closer to 14 minutes per mile.

So if you can't tell hard from easy based on distance and you can't tell hard from easy based on pace, what can you do? You can get yourself a heart rate monitor that won't lie to you. Instead, it will give you hard data.

Heart rate monitors (HRMs) measure your heart rate. They measure the number of beats per minute that your heart is beating in response to the demand being placed on it by your body. The HRM doesn't tell you how fast you are, how smart you are, or how rich you're going to be. It just tells you how fast your heart is beating.

Of course, some fancy units might also calculate the numbers of calories you're burning, the pace you are running, or even the distance you've travelled. But all calculate your heart rate.

And your heart is *your* heart. None of the numbers that you see on a HRM mean anything when compared to someone else's numbers. High numbers are not necessarily good, and low numbers aren't necessarily bad. Conversely, low numbers are not necessarily good and high numbers are not necessarily bad. The only number that matters to you is the one you're seeing.

The only way you'll know that you're getting into an honest-to-goodness training zone is by strapping on a monitor.

Effort-based training works. Everyone from the beginner to the world record holder has to understand the level of effort that his or her body can sustain, how much effort is not enough, how much is too much, and how to find that point of balance between doing enough to help and doing so much that it hurts.

Know Before You Go

You don't have to memorize complicated terms such as *cardiac reserve* in order to become a long-distance athlete. However, you do have to find a way to monitor your intensity as you train in order to last the entire distance. Purchase a heart rate monitor and use it during your training sessions. Besides helping you to stay in the zone, it will also provide you with feedback that can fuel your motivation.

Remember:

- Your heart is as unique to you as your fingerprints.
- Heart rate formulas don't work for the chronically fit.
- A heart rate monitor monitors your heart rate.
- Your heart rate is based on the demand placed on the heart.
- You cannot exceed your maximum heart rate.
- Your resting heart rate is the most important number.
- The number of beats available to train is your cardiac reserve.
- Your anaerobic threshold is the point at which you start to hear your breathing.

CHAPTER EIGHT

Choosing a Training Program

Too often, long-distance athletes choose training programs beyond their means. Yet in most cases, less is more and more is less. A little training goes a long way.

Mortal Dilemma: *I want to train hard and do well in the race, but I admit that I'm confused about which program I should choose. Which program is optimal for my goals, fitness level, and health history?*

In *Marathoning for Mortals*, we've included eight separate and unique training programs to help you reach the finish line safely and successfully. The programs vary depending on the length of your goal race (half-marathon vs. marathon) as well as how quickly you wish to finish that race. They range from walking the entire half-marathon to walking and running a marathon to running the entire marathon—and every variable in between.

Most important, always bear in mind that the best program is the one that best fits your personal inventory and goals.

The *Marathoning for Mortals* Training Programs

You can use one of eight different training programs to help you meet your goal. Four programs will train you to complete a half-marathon. Four others will train you to complete a full 26.2-mile marathon. For each race distance, the programs vary from walking the entire distance to running the distance.

No matter what type of runner you are or what type of goal you have, whether you simply want to finish the distance on the same day as you start or you want to run a personal best, you will find a program that meets your needs.

Each program schedule starts on a Monday and ends on a Sunday. Each workout falls on a specific day of the week for a specific reason. Each sequential session encourages your body to respond to the rhythm of progressively harder work, recovery, and adaptation.

That's why we've strategically mixed challenging training days with rest and cross-training days. This allows for optimal adaptation and recovery. Therefore, the sequence of workouts day to day is just as important as the intensity and duration.

If you need to modify your workouts, try to maintain the order of workouts from day to day.

To get a better idea of that order, let's take a look at the Run/Walk Half-Marathon training program. Specifically, let's look at week 1. The following is the effort-based sequence.

Monday	Tuesday	Wednesday	Thursday	Friday	Saturday	Sunday
Moderate	Moderate	Rest	Moderate	Moderate	Endurance	Rest

You'll notice that the pattern is two days "on," one day off, three days on, and one day off. Remember that the rest days are just as important as your long workout because they are when the training effect of recovery and gaining strength occurs. If you miss your workout on Tuesday, you still take a rest day on Wednesday.

This may not seem important in the early stages, but keep in mind that this is a long-distance training program. Your mileage and your intensity are going to increase as the weeks and months go on. You have to get it clear in your mind that the sequence is absolutely, positively sacred. If you miss a workout, it's gone forever. That's why you must choose a program that suits your lifestyle and that you can stick with over the long haul.

Mind Over Miles

When you glance at the programs, you may notice that you will never train the full distance of the race. For example, in all of the programs, the longest marathon training run equals 20 miles, and the longest half-marathon training run equals 10.

How can you expect your body to run for more than 26 miles if you've never run more than 20? How can you expect it to go for more than 13 when you've never run more than 10?

You'll have to place a certain amount of trust in our hands at this point, but we'll try to explain.

This is the great debate. How many miles does it take to optimally train for the half- and full marathons?

The great answer is: the number of miles that will prepare you rather than tear you. Train your body with quality, not quantity, and you will show up ready to race rather than injured, burnt out, or—worse—overtrained.

Still worried? We understand completely. John is a perfect example of why it is not necessary to walk, run, or even waddle the complete race distance in training. To date, he has run and walked

33 marathons and lots of half-marathons. Never once has he completed the race distance in training.

Do you want to know the secret? The recipe for success includes equal amounts of physical and mental strength. In every long-distance race, your body eventually gets tired and your mind must take over.

At the moment when your body begins to tire, you must make the conscious decision to think your way to the finish. Mental strength is the ability to focus on the task at hand and move your body as efficiently as possible to the final destination. Mental fitness is what will carry you past your training miles into the physical unknown.

You will become more mentally fit as the weeks progress in training. Your mind will see you through to new mile markers and challenging workouts. Your body and mind are equal partners, and together they will pave the way to a successful journey.

How to Pick the Best Program for You

To pick your program, sit down with the results of your personal inventory (from chapters 3 and 4) and match it with the program that makes the most sense. Although this may sound easy, there are many variables to review while making the decision. To help you navigate this process, we've described eight typical inventories as well as the training programs they match. Just match your personal inventory with one of the following participants, and voilà, you'll find the best training plan for you.

Walk Half-Marathon Training Program

Meet Mary. . . .

Mary was full of excitement and motivation to train for a long-distance race. She desperately wanted to complete the Disney Marathon and receive the Mickey Mouse Finisher's medal. She was determined to embark on the program that would take her there.

Then I looked over her health history and fitness regimen.

Mary admitted that she hadn't worked out in months. Even when she had worked out, her efforts were sporadic at best. She was 44 years old, had a history of back and knee pain, and was 35 pounds overweight.

I encouraged her to modify her goals. Mary began her quest for the Mickey Mouse medal by first *walking* a half-marathon. She has

---

Mortal Miracle

"I started running 4 years ago. Shortly after starting my walking training, I decided to try to run a little. I met with the group and ran with people whom I'd never met. I was shocked to know that I had run 7 miles! Two weeks later, I was diagnosed with thyroid cancer. The marathon was out—for that year. I couldn't believe it. I had gotten a taste of the marvelous feeling of running, and I just wouldn't stop.

"So I kept running. It empowered me. Unlike cancer, running made me feel good. It kept me in shape both physically and mentally. I learned that, through running, I was in charge of my body and gained strength not only in body, but also in mind and spirit. The long run gave me a freedom from reality. I ran the Philadelphia Distance Run just 2 weeks before my thyroid surgery and have run two since and also three Steamtown marathons! I'm hooked."

—Wendy, age 36

completed three races since and has progressed to walk/running her half-marathons. Mary hopes to eventually work up to the marathon distance.

You see, in the beginning, Mary's eyes were bigger than her stomach. Her goals extended quite a ways beyond her current state of health and fitness.

As with Mary, you, too, may need to start at a different place than you originally thought. That is okay because in the end you, like Mary, will progress without sabotage and with a healthy dose of personal success.

Is This Plan Right for You?

The Walk Half-Marathon program is a perfect place to start if you:

◆ Have a history of injury
◆ Are a few pounds overweight
◆ Have been inactive for many months

Walk/Run Half-Marathon Training Program

Meet Bob. . . .

Bob has been walking three or four times per week for 30 to 60 minutes for the past 13 months without injury or pain. However, he is running low on motivation to continue. He loves the benefits of walking but wants to add variety. That is why he decided to train for the Virginia Beach Half-Marathon.

Bob doesn't necessarily want to run continuously. Rather he wants to make his workouts more challenging with a combination of walking and running. He has tried to run, but every time he does, his efforts end in heavy breathing, frustration, and a few choice words.

Bob is 55 years old, healthy, and has a solid base of walking minutes under his belt. He could focus on speed walking but wants to work on sprinkling running into his regimen for something different. We both agreed the Walk/Run Half-Marathon training plan provided the best fit.

Bob is now 6 weeks into the Walk/Run program and loves it. He finds the program challenging yet manageable, as the program includes a higher ratio of walking minutes than running. He now feels highly motivated. He looks forward to completing the half-marathon and will do so with the smart walk/running system.

Is This Plan Right for You?

The Walk/Run Half-Marathon program is great for walkers who:

◆ Are looking to try running
◆ Have completed the half-marathon distance and want to improve their time

Run/Walk Half-Marathon Training Program

Meet Carol. . . .

Carol had been consistently running 30 to 45 minutes, three times per week, for 10 months. She set a goal to train to run the Indianapolis Mini Half-Marathon. She wanted to run the entire distance.

Carol had an on-and-off relationship with knee pain and was still trying to come back after having a baby 12 months earlier. She was 38 years old and about 20 pounds overweight. She hoped to lose those extra pounds by training for the race.

After a long heart-to-heart, I convinced Carol to train with the Run/Walk program. The Run/Walk was perfect for her. It included more running than walking, which allowed her body to withstand the impact of endurance training. Run/Walk also helped her lose weight more easily because she was able to complete the workouts without pain. She was even able to run stronger.

Carol finished the half-marathon in 2 hours—and lost 10 pounds training for it. She now can run continuously without pain, but she still includes the Run/Walk system in her regimen for recovery workouts.

Is This Plan Right for You?

The Run/Walk Half-Marathon program is perfect for:

◆ Runners who need a more forgiving strategy for long-distance training because of knee pain or an injury
◆ Walkers who want to integrate more running into their regimen
◆ Runners who want to safely increase distance without punishing their bodies
◆ Runners and walkers who need variety in their routines

Run Half-Marathon Training Program

Meet Tom. . . .

Tom ran four times per week on a treadmill at work for stress relief and to maintain his weight. Some buddies at work challenged Tom to run a marathon before his 40th birthday, which was 11 months away.

Tom was in good health but had never run more than 30 minutes in a workout. He had completed all of his runs indoors on a treadmill and at the same speed—10 minutes per mile. Tom was smart and elected to prepare for his first marathon by training for the Chicago Distance Classic half-marathon to build a strong mileage base and get race experience.

He was anxious to get started but was worried about running outdoors, especially once he reviewed the Run Half-Marathon plan and saw the endurance workouts.

We talked it over and came up with a compromise that would allow him to continue to train on a treadmill for some of the workouts while exploring the great outdoors for the others. He trained indoors during the week and outdoors for the endurance workout. This prepared him well for racing outdoors for the half-marathon and eventually the full marathon.

Tom was a smart runner. He was patient enough to properly build a gradual base of miles. He will successfully meet the challenge by his 40th birthday and probably be in the best shape of his life.

Is This Plan Right for You?

The Run Half-Marathon program is perfect for runners who:

◆ Want to run a complete half-marathon without walking
◆ Eventually want to run a full marathon but lack the training base to do so right away

Walk Marathon Training Program

Meet Stacey. . . .

Stacey had dreamed of traveling to Dublin, Ireland. When she found an opportunity to do so and help raise money for charity at the same time, she signed up as fast as she could. The Team in Training program offered her the chance to walk a marathon in Ireland while raising funds for research and patient aid for the Leukemia and Lymphoma Society.

Stacey was relatively active and had participated in group exercise classes two or three times per week at her gym. She wanted to finish the race, get in better shape, and lose weight. She was 32 years old, had no history of injury or illness, and was 50 pounds overweight.

Stacey followed the Walk Marathon training program. The program provided the tools to build her mileage base and focus on pace as well. Stacey had never participated in a race and was new to the sport of walking.

Little by little, Stacey adapted to the mileage, the lifestyle change, and the challenge of finishing—despite her friends and coworkers thinking she was out of her mind.

She proved she could do it on a cold, rainy day in Dublin. She had a goal, and the goal motivated her to walk regularly, raise more than $5,000 for Team in Training, and ultimately reach the finish line. She was so excited that she ran the last few steps to the finish with more energy than a 6-year-old.

Is This Plan Right for You?

The Walk Marathon program is perfect for those who:

◆ Are new to the marathon distance
◆ Are already relatively fit
◆ Have been exercising two or three times per week
◆ Are strongly motivated to finish the marathon distance

Walk/Run Marathon Training Program

Meet Susan. . . .

Susan had been walking for 3 years. She walked the Rock 'n' Roll Marathon in San Diego and finished it 2 minutes before the 8-hour cutoff time. She was the last walker to officially finish the race.

Susan set a goal to walk the Chicago Marathon but knew that she had to improve her time to meet the 7-hour cutoff. She had maintained a strong base of walking miles since the marathon and typically got in 3 to 5 miles three or four times per week. She was 47 and had knee pain while training for her first marathon. That knee pain has since subsided.

Susan agreed to train with the Walk/Run program. She quickly realized the benefits of sprinkling short minutes of running in her walking regimen. Her speed improved and she couldn't wait for the next training session.

She found that alternating walking with running challenged her and made the time go by quickly. She did a Walk/Run ratio of 3 to 1 (3 minutes of walking for every 1 minute of running) in the Chicago Marathon and finished in 6 hours and 55 minutes. She continues to walk/run in her everyday workouts and plans to someday complete another marathon.

Is This Plan Right for You?

The Walk/Run Marathon program is great for:

◆ Walkers who have a solid base but are seeking a challenge
◆ Runners who are getting back into running after an injury or a long expedition of couch surfing

Run/Walk Marathon Training Program

Meet John. . . .

John started training for a marathon because his friend Frank encouraged him to do so. Frank had been running for years, had completed several marathons, and wanted a running buddy. This was great for John. He had always wanted to run but lacked the motivation.

Frank had invited John to join him at a 5-K race. It was great fun for both of them even though Frank was much faster. They found races nearly every weekend, mostly 5-Ks and 10-Ks, and continued to run at the same races, but separately.

Once the goal become training for a marathon, everything changed. It wasn't so much a matter of cooperation; it was becoming a competition.

John struggled through his first few months of training. He had a difficult time keeping up with Frank and felt tired and sore most of the time. He enjoyed the feeling of accomplishment after each long run, but he couldn't understand why it wasn't getting easier. John was training hard, but he struggled to finish the workouts. He was 30, healthy, and in shape. Why wasn't he progressing?

It didn't take long before John developed a stubborn case of knee pain. His physical therapist recommended time off and cross-training. Although he followed her advice, it took more than a month to recover, and he missed the marathon.

John decided to take another shot and train for the Marine Corps Marathon. This time he followed the Run/Walk program. He progressed without injury and even improved his speed. He ran so well that he passed his buddy Frank at the 22-mile marker in the marathon.

John learned that it pays to be patient and build a sound foundation. John checked his ego at the door and learned from his mistakes. He took a different road on his journey but reached the same destination in less time!

Is This Plan Right for You?

The Run/Walk Marathon program is perfect for:

◆ Runners who are injured or have suffered injuries in the past
◆ Those who have been running for less than a year and don't have a base of at least 20 miles per week
◆ Walk/runners who want a new challenge
◆ Veteran runners looking for an alternate strategy for improving speed and performance

Run Marathon Training Program

Meet Shannon. . . .

Shannon ran her first marathon last year and has since set a goal to improve her time at the New York City Marathon. Shannon is 27 years old, has always been active playing sports and running, and has rarely been injured.

Although Shannon finished her first marathon, she struggled to complete the last 6 miles and wants to run the entire marathon at a strong and even pace. Her legs cramped at 21 miles and she managed to crawl the last few miles to earn her medal.

In reviewing her past training program, we both agreed she was training too hard. She was running 5 out of 7 days of the week. Her pace was too fast. She didn't give herself enough time to recover. Therefore, when she asked her body to perform on race day, her body calmly replied with a set of nasty hamstring cramps.

Shannon trained with the Run program the second time around, but this time she decreased her frequency, cross-trained twice per week, and rested more during the week as well as throughout the training program.

Shannon completed the New York City Marathon without muscle cramping and with a huge smile on her face. This time, she enjoyed every step and felt strong during the entire race. She took our advice and walked 1 minute at every aid station, took time to get the fluids in her body rather than on her body, and bettered her time by 8 minutes.

Is This Plan Right for You?

The Run Marathon program is perfect for:

◆ First-time marathoners with a base of at least 20 miles per week for at least 6 months

◆ First-time marathoners who are injury-free

◆ Veteran runners who are struggling to race without injuries or whose times are slipping

Unique Programs for Your Unique Body

Achieving a goal starts with a realistic plan. Begin with a realistic program based on your health history and progress from there. Set your goal to finish the race comfortably and enjoyably rather than torturing yourself until your body quits.

With this in mind, if you find yourself struggling to get in the training workouts, you are most likely in a program that is too difficult. It doesn't mean that you can never train with this program; it simply means that you will need to prepare with a different program to get where you want to go. Anyone can beat their body to a pulp to reach a destination, but it takes wisdom and patience to get there and enjoy the process.

Train smart and modify your program to meet your current fitness level. Listen to your body, follow a realistic program, and day by day, week by week, your body will appreciate your intelligent choice and reward you by working with you and adapting.

Know Before You Go

Before moving on to Part Three, look over your personal inventory and try to match your answers to one of our fictional inventories. Then carefully consider and pick the best training plan for you. Remember to base your choice on your fitness background and lifestyle, not on lofty goals or peer pressure. Also, if the going feels rough after the first few weeks, reconsider your choice. You may need to switch to a different plan.

Remember:

- The training programs are sequential.
- Choose a program based on your personal inventory.

- Don't choose a program that is beyond you.
- Reaching for the stars is fine until your arms get tired.
- You can change programs if you need or want to.
- No program is right for everyone.
- Only you can decide which program you want to follow.
- The programs are only as good as you make them.
- The wrong program is worse than no program.
- When in doubt, be conservative.

Part Three

The
Toolbox

Everything you need to take

the journey of a lifetime

CHAPTER NINE

Injury Prevention

"No pain, no gain" has been the exercise mantra for generations of athletes. Unfortunately, for the adult-onset athlete, "No pain, no gain" is also the formula for injury, disappointment, and failure.

Mortal Dilemma: *I've had aches and pains while I train, most of which subside in a few days. How do I determine when the soreness is an early sign of injury or a normal response to the training progression?*

Not too long ago, I, John, could have been the poster child for training stupidity. I come from a generation in which boys learned to take it like a man, in which our heroes were forever getting shot up—with bullets and cortisone—and in which playing hurt was the gold standard for dedication. I also come from a generation that created the need for hip and knee replacements because we wore ours out.

So the first sign of an injury was a badge of honor for me. I actually felt excited the first time I had to go to an orthopedic doctor.

I had a sports injury. I was going to see someone who specialized in treating injured athletes. What could be better?

In a bizarre way, I even felt excited as I sat on the examination table for the first time. After all, a *sports* doctor was examining me. He was trying to find the source and cause of an *athletic* injury. Better yet, it was an injury that I had given myself. This was no accidental injury. This was on purpose. This must mean that I—a former couch potato—was now a true athlete.

As if I needed to prove my abject ignorance, I brought in a printout of my training schedule from the previous year. Not only was I injured, but I also had the evidence! I showed the doctor exactly when I'd increased my mileage too much and done too much speed work. I pointed to the date on which I ran instead of taking the day off.

I thought he would be impressed with the details of my training. I was wrong. He didn't see the journal of an athlete in my hands. He saw a litany of training errors and bullheadedness. Rather than congratulating me on my toughness, he chastised me for my foolhardiness.

I was shocked.

Still, I had been selected in the lottery for the 100th running of the Boston Marathon and I was bound and determined to run it. That first visit ended with a cortisone shot in the knee. The pain, I will tell you now, was excruciating. Yet even then, I felt a sick satisfaction in knowing that I was suffering the pain of an athlete.

The second visit started with a little more tension between the good doctor and me. I didn't mention that I had pulled out of a marathon 6 weeks earlier because I couldn't take the pain in my knee. I didn't mention that I had run marathons two weekends in a row and then run a half-marathon two weeks later. I didn't mention that I had limped through a 16-mile training run that very week. I just told him that the knee was acting up again and that I had to run the London Marathon in a few weeks.

He was terse. He would give me another shot, but that was it—no more. I couldn't keep hammering my knees and expecting him to put me out of my pain. I told him that I understood, took the shot, and ran the marathon.

The next time he found me sitting on the examination table, he didn't even pretend to listen to my excuses. He told me straight out that I was training like I was 25 years old even though I was nearly 50. Game over. No more shots. No more pills. And if I didn't get smarter soon, there'd be no more running.

The Lesson Behind the Injury

It didn't occur to me that running could be an addiction as hard to control as alcohol, cigarettes, or drugs. It should have seemed clear to me early on. After all, at various times in my life, I'd been addicted to alcohol, cigarettes, and drugs. Why wouldn't I apply the same addictive behavior to my running?

I would, and I did. I kept running even when I knew that the worst thing I could do was run. I ran when I was sick, just as I had smoked when I had a cold. It was hard to do, but that didn't stop me.

I ran farther than was healthy, just as I had drunk more than was healthy. I ran too far and too hard just to get the buzz from the runner's high just as surely as I had popped pills to get high. Running became just another excuse to abuse my body.

Of course, on the surface, running was a good thing. It was a healthy obsession, a healthy alternative to the booze and cigarettes. It was also the perfect way to stay totally separated from my body.

For those of us who come to running a little later in life, it's easy to think that we can apply the same skills and temperament that we've used in every other part of our lives. We can't. The drive, obsession, compulsion, or misplaced discipline that made us either successful or addicted has no place in a rational, thoughtful training program.

Running injury-free, for me, starts with getting my head on straight. Running and walking have to become things with positive outcomes, not negative ones. I've got to learn enough about my body and my personality to construct, modify, and stay with a training program that gets me to the starting line first and the finish line second.

Running injury-free means that my ego has to take a backseat to my rational brain. The child in me who thinks that missing a day of running means I'm lazy and undisciplined has to yield to the adult athlete in me who says that some days the best training I can do is to rest.

The Top Three Running Injuries

Okay, here goes. We're going to talk about injuries. Before we start, understand that we didn't try to describe every possible running-related injury with the attendant treatment and cure. Whole books have been written on such a topic. Rather, we've simply created a primer, a quick and dirty explanation of what can happen, what might happen, and what to do if it happens.

In all the years that we've been at this, with all the new athletes that we've coached or advised, the vast majority of running-related complaints come down to these three.

- ◆ Iliotibial band syndrome (IT band syndrome)
- ◆ Chondromalacia patellae (runner's knee)
- ◆ Plantar fasciitis (PF)

Mortal Miracle

"At age 52 it's hard to have the muscle power, energy, and enthusiasm to finish an entire marathon. After all, middle age changes not only your body, but also your mind. I've learned that I don't need to go for the gusto—the whole marathon—to feel good about myself. Training for the half-marathon is just about right for those of us who need a little more recovery time and less impact on our tired old bones."

—Becky, age 52

With a little practice you'll actually be able to pronounce "iliotibial (ILL-ee-oh-tib-ee-al) band syndrome," but you might as well just say "IT band syndrome." And "chondromalacia patellae" will never roll off your lips, so get used to saying "runner's knee." Whatever you call these injuries, they may very well become a part of your life if you're not careful.

The IT band is actually a large, wide tendon that stretches about 60 feet from just below the outside of your knee to somewhere deep inside your butt. Okay, maybe not 60 feet, but it really does go on a long way. The pain is almost always a fairly specific point a few inches below the bend in your leg. The pain can be dull most of the time and become acute when you start to walk or run.

IT band syndrome is common among all runners but even more common among women. The angle between a woman's hip and knee (called the Q angle) is greater than it is for men. The result is that the IT band tends to get stretched tighter across the outside of the knee joint in women than it does in men. But many, many men find themselves with IT band syndrome as well.

IT band syndrome does not normally just appear. It usually begins as a nagging kind of pain that seems more like an inconvenience than a true injury. In fact, IT band syndrome can be so subtle at first that you might actually continue to train and convince yourself (as I did) that it is actually getting better despite the fact that you continue to aggravate it.

This is the great danger of IT band syndrome because it doesn't just suddenly rear its ugly head. It starts out as a dull ache that you can train through for a while, and then eventually the pain gets so intense that you have to stop. The bad news is that by the time it gets to that point, you've greatly extended your recovery time.

The IT band runs alongside the knee bone to help keep things stable. If you fatigue your muscles, they can't keep the band in place and it starts rubbing against the bone like a rope on a rock. Every step makes it worse. The only cure is rest.

Chondromalacia patellae, or runner's knee, is another common overuse injury that affects many new long-distance athletes. And in case you were wondering, walkers do get runner's knee. Technically, runner's knee is an inflammation in the cartilage under the kneecap. When that cartilage gets inflamed, the kneecap, or patella, can't slide up and down through its normal motion.

Like IT band syndrome, runner's knee is not a traumatic injury. It doesn't happen instantly. It comes on slowly, sometimes over as long as a year. You'll know it's runner's knee if the pain is isolated underneath the kneecap. It will also get worse during activity, when you go down stairs or hills, or sometimes after you sit with your knee bent. If it gets severe enough, you can sometimes actually hear the cartilage crackling.

Runner's knee is caused by weak quadriceps muscles that fail to anchor the patella in place. Instead the patella tracks incorrectly, causing friction. As painful as it is, it is also completely curable and preventable.

Runner's knee is nearly always the result of doing too many miles too soon. If you build your mileage gradually so that your quadriceps get stronger along with your calves and hamstring muscles, you can avoid the pain and frustration. And as with IT band syndrome, you cannot train through the pain.

The final jewel is plantar fasciitis. The plantar tendon runs underneath your foot and connects at the heel and near the ball of your foot. As this tendon tightens under the stress of running, it pulls the bone of the heel forward and down. This hurts. The pain associated with PF is nearly always felt in the heel. It's that sharp pain that you get when you take the first step out of bed in the morning. PF usually subsides as the day goes on. It doesn't go away, but it does get better.

That's the biggest danger with PF. You can get fooled into thinking that it's temporary. I've known people who have suffered with PF for years only to end up with a heel spur that requires much more serious intervention.

PF is most often brought on by running too many miles before you're ready. It takes time for your feet to develop the strength to remain stable and to support themselves under the stress of running and walking long distances. They will get stronger if you give them time.

PF can also be caused by wearing a shoe that doesn't bend where your foot does. Look at your bare foot. Now wiggle your toes and see where it bends. It will bend up near the ball of the foot, not in the middle of your foot. If you grab your current pair of shoes (running, walking, or casual) and notice that they bend anywhere other than at the ball of the foot, you are asking for trouble.

The good news about PF is that it often responds very well to a quick and relatively inexpensive solution. For a fair number of

Mortal Miracle

"At age 52, I've been running for just over 12 years and marathoning for almost 6. I've completed 41 marathons so far.

"I had taken up running as a way to 'get in shape' for church basketball. A friend of mine—Steve, a runner 10 years younger than me—said, 'You've got a 40th birthday coming up; why don't you run a 10-K to celebrate?' I said, 'Sure. What's a 10-K?' It went from there.

"I had three goals: One, finish. Two, run the whole way. Three, not get passed by anyone over 70 in the first mile. I accomplished all three, getting passed by a 73-year-old at mile 1.5 and a 10-year-old at mile 2! But I finished and was happy. I ran 57:57 and had *no* idea what that time meant, good or bad.

"A couple of weeks later, I got the race results booklet in the mail and found that the winner in my age group had beaten me by nearly 20 minutes! I went to my friend Steve and said, 'I can never get that much faster. Maybe 10 minutes, but not 20!' 'Ron,' my wise friend said, 'You aren't racing against *his* time. You will be racing next time against *your* time. That is what it is all about—how to better yourself.'

"He was right. If I had tried to cut off those 20 minutes I would have overtrained, probably gotten hurt, and definitely gotten discouraged and quit. But instead, I have—each day since—gone out and seen what I can do compared to what the day offers *me*, at *my* ability and *my* pace."

—Ron, age 52

long-distance athletes, simply replacing the standard insole that comes with most new shoes will clear up the problem almost immediately. These replacement insoles generally offer more arch support than ones that come standard with shoes. More arch support takes pressure off your plantar tendon. Replacement insoles—brands like Superfeet, Spenco, and Softsole—are available at running specialty stores.

That's our top three. With luck and patience, you'll never have to deal with any of them. But if you are not so patient and not so lucky, you'll need to know a few additional things to help you get through the frustration of an injury.

The Care and Feeding of the Body

Unless you've recently arrived from the planet Xenon, you've probably heard about RICE therapy. No, not long grain and steamed rice—RICE rice: rest, ice, compression, and elevation. With all the advances in medical treatment, with all the miracle drugs on the market, for the most common injuries there's still nothing that works better than rest, ice, compression, and elevation.

R is for REST. At the onset of an injury—notice the word *onset*—stop what you're doing and rest. Nothing good is going to happen if you keep training with an injury. Our own rule of thumb is to take 3 days off. Three days. Three full days. That means if it hurts on Monday, you take Tuesday, Wednesday, and Thursday off and see how it feels on Friday. (We know you. You figure if it hurts on Monday, that's one day. Then Tuesday is a second day and Wednesday is the third, so you can run on Thursday. Not.)

In many cases, the inflammation that was causing the pain will subside substantially in 3 days. If it doesn't, take 3 more days off. If it still hurts, it's time to get professional help.

I is for ICE. Whether you suffer a traumatic injury, like a sprained ankle, or an overuse injury, like those we just described, get ice on the affected area as soon as possible. The sooner you get ice on an injury, the sooner you will stop the inflammation response and the sooner you will begin to heal and recover.

Keep ice on the injury for about 10 to 20 minutes. What you're trying to do is (1) get the inflammation to subside and (2) get the blood vessels to constrict. After 20 minutes, take the ice away and let the area warm up completely. This will encourage increased blood flow, which will speed up the healing and recovery.

Repeat this cycle of ice/warmup a few times, and try to do it two or three times a day for the 3 days that you are *resting*.

C is for COMPRESSION. Compression works best for acute injuries, such as ankle sprains. Wrapping your ankle as soon as you sprain it will squeeze out inflammation, preventing fluids from accumulating in your ankle and causing pain and stiffness. However, for the vast majority of overuse injuries, you need to get to the root of the problem and solve it. Compression only provides a short-term solution.

E is for ELEVATION. Again, for us as distance athletes, the kind of injuries we're most likely to face won't require elevation. Again, sprained ankles provide the most obvious exception.

Five Things You Can Do to Prevent Injuries

Even experienced athletes and coaches get injured.

—ॐ—

I, Jenny, stepped into a hole and sprained my ankle on the first day of the 2001 Eco-Challenge in New Zealand. We had 7 days and more than 300 miles to go, and I wasn't about to quit. I should have, make no mistake. So I, too, am susceptible to my enthusiasm outwitting my coach's wisdom.

But through the experience, I came to understand the value of physical therapy. After the race, I spent 2 months healing and 4 months building strength. Thanks to the help of Alex McKinney, a physical therapist, I walked away from the experience a better athlete and coach. Alex knew what I was going through and how to help. He is a Boston-qualified marathoner, an Ironman Triathlete, and director of the Athletico Sports Medicine Endurance Program. He taught me to detect my weaknesses and balance my strengths. I was so impressed with my rehab experience at Athletico that I asked Alex to share a few of his tips for long-distance athletes. Here's what he had to say.

1. Listen to your body. Aches and pains that persist longer than 3 or 4 days are red flags. Take a few days off and cross-train with an activity that doesn't aggravate your condition. Do this until the ache subsides.

Then gradually progress your miles and modify the distances to increase no more than 10 percent each week. That means that if your total mileage last week equaled 10 miles, your mileage this week should total no more than 11 miles.

2. Stretch. Flexibility is the most overlooked component of training. Tight muscles lead to muscle imbalances and eventually injuries. Regular stretching will improve your muscle and joint flexibility, which will directly improve your gait and form as well as help you prevent injuries. Include stretching at the end of your workout after your cooldown.

Hold each stretch for 30 seconds—no bouncing—hitting each muscle group from your shoulders to your calves.

3. Strength train and cross-train. Include regular strength training and cross-training in your routine to maintain muscular balance. When strength training, focus on the muscles in your core (abdomen and low back), hips, pelvis, and legs.

4. Consult a running specialty store professional when purchasing shoes. Replace your shoes every 300 to 500 miles or every 6 months, whichever comes first.

5. Use your common sense. Follow a realistic training program that is based on your health and exercise history.

How to Rehabilitate an Injury

So what do you do if, despite doing everything right, you still get injured?

It happens—even to the best of us. Distance athletes' injuries are typically overuse injuries, meaning that the body does not have the ability or time to repair the tissue breaking down during the activity. For some injuries, you may be able to continue to train. For others, you should take a week or more off from running.

To figure out how much—if any—downtime you need, determine the severity of your injury.

◆ Type I: pain after activity only
◆ Type II: pain during and after activity, but not severe enough to make you cut short a workout
◆ Type III: pain during activity so severe that you quit early
◆ Type IV: chronic, unremitting pain that makes you want to surgically remove a part of your body

You can continue to run with Type I or II pain, as long you understand and address what's causing the symptoms (e.g., tight calves causing posterior leg pain) and as long as your pain does not intensify. Listen to your body. Don't wait until Type III or IV pain to adjust or get help. Waiting may result in time off from training or end your running career altogether.

Seek professional medical help if you have Type II, III, or IV pain or any type of pain that does not go away after 4 days of active or complete rest. Consult running or athletic professionals, as they will be open to guiding you back on course. Doctors who don't run often will simply tell you not to run. So seek out a podiatrist, an orthopedist, or a physical therapist who runs. You can find these professionals by asking around at specialty running or walking stores, reading regional athletic newspapers or magazines, and by asking your friends who run.

Know Before You Go

Before you move on to the next chapter, do a quick body scan. Does anything hurt? During your next workout, do the same. Mentally scan your body from head to toe and hone in on pain, aches, tightness, or discomfort. Learning to tune into your body's subtle messages is one of the most important tricks to preventing injuries. Remember:

- No pain, *your* gain.
- It's never smart to do something stupid.
- Don't be a hero. If it hurts, stop.
- Injuries don't just go away; they have to heal.
- Today's ache can be tomorrow's injury.
- Pain is your body's way of saying you're doing too much.
- Nearly every injury responds well to rest.
- When in doubt, ice the injury.
- Listening to your body means listening to your body.
- Don't try to make up for missed training by doing more.

CHAPTER TEN

Cross-Training

By adding other activities like cycling, rowing, and strength training to your program, you can get stronger and fitter and have fun learning new skills.

Mortal Dilemma: *I like running and walking. I understand why I need to increase my mileage, work on my form, and even try to increase my speed. Why isn't just doing what I'm doing enough?*

—⁓—

Nearly everything I've discovered about my nonrunning male penguin self began as a cross-training exercise. When it became clear that I couldn't continue to put in the miles I was running week after week, I bought a mountain bike and headed for the trails. That led to learning how to paddle a canoe and kayak, which led to getting into the outdoors, which led to hiking and trekking.

Cross-training has allowed me to find out what I like and what I don't. It has allowed me to define myself in broader terms than just "runner." Make no mistake that running and walking are and will always be my core aerobic activities, but cross-training activi-

ties have helped me to create a more comprehensive athletic pro-
file and a stronger, more balanced body.

In addition to those benefits, cross-training offers an aerobic
outlet for those recovering from running injuries, and I've had
plenty of those. Fortunately, I've discovered that there's almost no
limit to what you can do other than running in order to maintain
your aerobic base.

The good news is that if you use a set of muscles over and over,
they'll eventually get stronger. That bad news is that if you use a set
of muscles over and over, they may also wear down. The key to a
successful long-distance training program is building the strength
you need while protecting yourself from overuse and injury. One
of the best ways to do that is by cross-training.

I began my life as an athlete by riding a bicycle. Later I discovered that I really enjoyed running. Later still, when a friend invited
me to participate in a triathlon, I learned how to swim. I was excited about being a multisport athlete. It never occurred to me that
I was cross-training. I was just having a good time doing three different activities every week.

A funny thing happened shortly after my first triathlon. I ran
my fastest 5-K ever. As it turns out, a little less running and a little
more biking and swimming actually made me a better and faster
runner. Mixing in nonrunning activities allowed me to spend more
time active every week without feeling sore as a result. And as a new
athlete, I was eager to do anything that would allow me to be more
active. So for me, cross-training isn't a burden; it's a blessing.

Which cross-training activities you choose depends on your
personal tastes and interests. I've always enjoyed riding a bicycle, so
that was an easy choice. I had a good friend who, for reasons
known only to him, really enjoyed pounding away on a stairclimber. In fact—just to give you an insight into his psyche—he

once trained for a marathon using only the stairclimber. He never ran one step on the roads and he did pretty well.

How you cross-train isn't as important as the fact that you do cross-train. A change of pace and a change of place every week will create a welcome break from your training routine.

Coach Jenny and I have compiled the following list of our top 10 cross-training activities. These happen to be our favorites, and ones that are the most accessible to us. They may be right for you, or you may discover others. It doesn't matter. One or all of these activities can benefit your training. Just find a convenient activity that you enjoy.

Bicycling

I've already mentioned that I like to ride my bike. It started when I was a kid. I felt a freedom and sense of exploration when I got on the bike. I still feel it today. These days I spend most of my time riding a mountain bike. About half of the time I can actually get off-road. The rest of the time, I ride on a path or street.

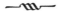

Like John, I loved to ride a bike as a kid. I started riding just as soon as my feet could reach the Big Wheel pedals. My racing career started by challenging all the boys on the block to a Big Wheel race. I turned my Big Wheel in for a brand-new, powder blue Schwinn bike. This was the big time. It had a flowered banana seat, long sparkled blue and silver streamers on the bar ends, and an orange flag to top it all off.

Because cycling offers a nonimpact activity that targets op- posing muscle groups, it perfectly complements your running and walking program. Whether inside on a stationary cycle or outside on your bike, cycling trains the cardiovascular system without adding more stress by impact.

Stairclimbing

As I, John, mentioned, I had a friend who loved the stairclimber. In fact, he developed entire routines, which included turning around and facing backward on the machine. You can image the looks he got from the less fit folks in the gym.

I've always viewed that stair machine as a low-risk, low-impact method of getting my heart rate up without taking any chances with my joints. You can do a solid session on the stair machine at a very high level of effort without much danger of injury.

Climbing the staircases in buildings never had much appeal to me, but the wife of a good friend and *Runner's World* colleague who is an ultra runner has been known to haunt hotel staircases late at night. It can be a great substitute for hill work if you've got the nerve.

When the first stairclimbing machine was introduced, I thought it was just a form of medieval torture. It was called the Gauntlet, and as I stepped up to program the time, I knew I was in for a challenging workout. As the steps began to rotate round and round, I quickly learned that if I didn't keep up, the machine would eject me halfway across the room. In a Lucille Ball moment, I began to lose pace and found myself doing nothing short of crawling to stay on the machine. I started too fast and couldn't keep up with the stairs. Everyone in the gym enjoyed the circus performance. Times have changed. Now machines include emergency stop buttons. Imagine that.

Stairclimbing, either on a machine or in a stairwell, offers a beneficial form of active rest. Some machines include upper body movement, and though they require a little more coordination, these machines provide additional benefits because they call in the help of your upper body and actively discourage the "lean and climb" technique. (This is when you crank up the speed of the stairs and then lean on the bars because you can't keep up.)

Elliptical Training

Elliptical what? Precor was the first company to develop a machine that combines the movements of the treadmill with stair-climbing and cross-country skiing. Though it sounds complex,

Mortal Miracle

"I quit smoking almost 2 years ago and started walking with my dog. Eventually I figured I'd try running, adding 1 minute at a time. The day I went from running 1 minute to 2 minutes, I thought my lungs would explode and my head would pop off. But I made it. Eight months later I ran my first half-marathon, and I'm planning to finish my third in 2 weeks.

"These days, I run every other day, I ride my bike to the climbing gym, I hike, and I climb mountains. I know I can do anything I set my mind to, because I can run 21.1 kilometers. Running is powerful and I am hooked."

—Meg, age 32

the elliptical trainer provides one of the best forms of cross-training because it eliminates impact and includes forward and reverse elliptical motion.

When you're "running" on the trainer, you feel as if you're floating. It's a great way to rehab an overuse injury without impact to the muscles, tendons, and joints. Moving your legs forward simulates running and walking and requires your core muscles, hips, and legs to work together.

Moving in reverse focuses on the muscles in your gluteus and hamstrings, which are solely responsible for pulling the leg down and through the running and walking stride. Consider elliptical training a low-impact alternative to running and walking, one that can help you train all of the muscles in the lower body.

Rowing and Paddling

Whether rowing indoors on a machine or kayaking or rowing outdoors on the water, you'll discover a world unlike anything in the running world. Paddling is like running or walking with your upper body. If done correctly, you will use your core muscles as primary movers and your arms, hips, and legs as secondary assistants.

You can go places by way of water and see nature that you otherwise would never see from land. And at the gym, the rowing machine is almost always open. No waiting on line to get in a workout. If we're not careful, the secret will be exposed. We'll head to the gym only to find every rower in motion and then to Lake Michigan only to see the water covered by a sea of kayaks!

The rewards to taking the risk and paddling on water are plentiful. We've paddled on Resurrection Bay in Alaska and seen endangered bald eagles, made our way down a scenic river in Kauai,

Hawaii, and rode the rapids in West Virginia. Paddling and kayaking offer a nonimpact activity that can be recreational or competitive. For the purpose of cross-training, keep it fun.

Swimming

As I mentioned, I spent several of my early years as an athlete participating in triathlons. The swimming section was always the most difficult for me, but also—in some ways—the most satisfying. That is, until I saw a photo of myself standing in a cold lake wearing a Speedo. I gave up triathlons after that.

Swim training can provide either a relaxing and refreshing experience or a heart-pounding, air-sucking workout. Either way it offers a completely nonimpact vacation for land-based training. I found swimming the most fun when I viewed it as an escape from my land-based training and just let myself swim laps.

If you are struggling with aches and pains, water training provides a safe alternative to active recovery that will maintain your cardiovascular fitness.

Water Running and Walking

All of us would improve our form if we spent some time running in water. Because water is much heavier than air, it makes all those little "hitches in our get-a-longs" become very obvious. Unfortunately, most of us don't grab the aqua vest until we're injured.

I spent several weeks one year doing all of my training in the deep end of the pool. I did easy runs, speed work, and even a few long runs without ever having my feet touch solid ground. Other than the smell of chlorine on my skin and hair, I found the experiences very rewarding.

I learned about the benefits of water running, however, by necessity. I completed the Chicago Marathon and ended up with a stress fracture in my heel. For recovery I tried training with a small group of five runners in the deep end of the pool on Monday, Wednesday, and Friday mornings at 6 A.M. I couldn't think of anything worse than having to wake up at 4:30 A.M. to work out in a cold pool. But I gave it a try and actually improved my cardiovascular fitness. And my heel recovered.

You can water train in the shallow end of the pool with your feet touching the bottom or with the help of an aqua vest in the deep end of the pool. (You can purchase these vests specifically designed for pool running at most sports stores.) The deeper you go, the more water resistance you encounter and the more challenging the workout. Water running creates a nonimpact, moderate- to high-intensity workout that can help you heal from an injury or give your muscles a timeout from the impact of land training.

Yoga and Pilates

Guys: Don't skip this section. Yoga and Pilates are *not* "chick" activities. You'd know that if you had been in the Pilates class with me that was led by a 60ish-year-old woman who was meaner, tougher, and nastier than any drill sergeant I've ever encountered.

Yoga provides a great way to increase your overall flexibility without having to think about stretching, and Pilates builds your core strength like nothing else. Both types of classes, whether taught at a gym or on video, provide unique alternatives to distance training. They will challenge you in ways unforeseen and provide a low-stress resource for building core strength and balanced flexibility.

Strength Training

In the years when I, John, had easy access to a gym, I used to strength train at least 3 days a week. Oddly enough, it was during those same years that I had some of my greatest triumphs as an athlete. Go figure.

Building muscle balance front-to-back and side-to-side is important for everyone, but it is especially important to those in the early stages of their running careers. You are coming to these running programs with the body that you developed more by chance than by good planning. Strength training can help make your body a better tool to help you achieve your goals.

We're not talking about building bulk like the Incredible Hulk, but rather lean muscle tissue that will help you in the long run. A regular strength program in the form of power yoga, Pilates, Nautilus machines, calisthenics, or free weights will build a solid foundation that will support you in any weather condition. A strong body will help maintain proper form as you add miles and speed to your running.

A long-distance athlete's strength program should vary depending on the season. While training for a race, include strength training twice per week with at least 2 days in between. You can do strength workouts on short-distance training workout days or cross-training days. Always do it at least 2 days before your endurance workout. Include all the major muscle groups in the upper body, lower body, and core.

Before or after your "in-season" training program, you can boost your strength sessions to 3 days per week. Because strength training breaks down muscle fibers and creates microscopic tears, you must allow 48 hours between each workout for your muscles to fully recover.

During each exercise, go to the point of fatigue or momentary muscular failure. Don't let the sound of that scare you. It means only that you should lift to the point at which you can no longer lift the weight with good form. You should reach this point within 8 to 12 repetitions. If you can't lift the weight eight times, it is too heavy. Conversely, if you can lift the weight all day, it is way too light.

Group Exercise Classes

Like many women my age, I first became interested in fitness when Jane Fonda developed her home video. I remember lying on my back with my feet over my head, stretching out after an hour and a half of dancing, skipping, and jumping in my leg warmers. I knew the video so well that I could follow it without even seeing it, and I would sing along with Jane. Perhaps this had something to do with me learning how to teach aerobics and step classes. Ah, those were the good old days.

There are tons of classes now: high impact, low impact, step, spinning, Jazzercise, funk, cardio boxing, and even strip aerobics. The options are endless and offer something for everyone.

Hiking and Trekking

If there's one hidden benefit of being a runner or walker, it would be that it allows you—heck, it encourages you to get out and see the world with your own two feet. From the Na Pali coastline on Kauai to Mount Baker in Washington State, we've experienced the world in a way we never knew possible.

Hiking, or trekking as some like to call it, requires every muscle to stay vertical on uneven and, most times, mountainous terrain. The uneven terrain challenges the stabilizing muscles in our feet, legs, and hips while the hills or mountains build a strong muscular and cardiovascular system—all of this while being in the great outdoors. Your efforts are always rewarded with a great view. You just can't beat it.

You'll even find toys that can improve your balance over technical terrain and train your upper body in the process. Trekking poles are the latest fad in hiking and quickly turn us two-legged humans into four-legged ones. You can hike anywhere in your hometown on grass or paths or on vacation in state or national parks. It doesn't matter where you hike; just get out and enjoy the great outdoors.

Top Five Reasons to Cross-Train During Long-Distance Training

Cross-training supplements and balances your long-distance training program. Find activities you enjoy and you will soon reap the benefits.

To fully convince you of the benefits of cross-training, we enlisted the help of our friend, triathlon and swimming coach Mike Norman of Chicago Endurance Sports. Mike spends his days teaching athletes the benefits of cross-training. He was kind enough to share his secrets with us. According to Mike, cross-training:

1. Improves running/walking performance. Strengthening your nonrunning and nonwalking muscles through cross-training will improve your ability to maintain proper running form in the later stages of the race. This will make you a more efficient runner overall. You will also benefit from increased stability on uneven terrain.

2. Improves recovery. By focusing on nonrunning and non-walking activities, you reduce the strain on your distance training-specific muscles and connective tissue. This will allow those muscles to fully recover before your next distance workout.

3. Increases overall fitness. You will be able to perform a variety of activities instead of just running or walking. Everyday tasks such as lifting heavy items, carrying children, and climbing stairs will be easier, too. You may even burn more total calories, so you can also increase fat loss.

4. Reduces risk of injury. Every time you perform a distance training workout, you put a lot of strain on your leg muscles. Even short workouts can put excess stress on already sore, tired muscles, and your risk of injury increases. Cross-training allows you to get in a workout without adding more stress to your leg muscles.

5. Makes you happy. Cross-training allows you to add variety to your training to avoid boredom and burnout. You can take a break from the structure of your training and have some fun doing something different.

Top Five Reasons to Cross-Train After the Party Is Over

After you've completed your marathon or half-marathon, cross-training provides a crucial ingredient for your mental and physical recovery. Here are some important reasons to cross-train after your big day.

1. Mental recovery. It's not uncommon for distance athletes to feel depressed after completing a race of this distance. It took a lot of commitment and effort to train for and compete in the race. Cross-training helps fill the void, gives you a break from the routine, and helps rejuvenate your mind.

2. Physical recovery. Your muscles are extremely vulnerable during the first few weeks following a half-marathon or marathon. Jumping right back in to an intense distance training schedule can delay your recovery. Cross-training will allow your distance muscles time to recover while still maintaining your fitness level.

3. No postrace weight gain. It's very easy to be complacent during the first few weeks after your race, and it's all too easy to gain a few unwanted pounds. Cross-training is a fun way to help burn those extra calories and maintain the fitness you've worked so hard to achieve.

4. Social benefits. Here's your chance to meet new people and try new activities. You may find some new training partners who share your next big training goal or you may discover a sport that you may not have even considered trying before. Enjoy and explore!

5. Simply put, it's fun!

Know Before You Go

Before moving on to chapter 11, consider some ways—other than running and walking—that you might enjoy moving your body. Plan to embark on one type of cross-training activity at least once a week. Remember:

- Don't add cross-training. Substitute it for other workouts.
- Cross-training builds the muscles that running and walking don't.
- Any cross-training is better than no cross-training.
- Find an activity that you enjoy, and you'll stick with it.
- Learn one new activity a year.

- You don't have to get good at something to enjoy it.
- Buy the equipment you need so that you're more likely to stick with cross-training.
- Cross-training improves your performance.
- Cross-training speeds your recovery.
- Cross-training improves your overall fitness.

CHAPTER ELEVEN

Nutrition

We've all heard the expression "You are what you eat." If that were the case, many of us would look like hot fudge sundaes. Just changing your view of what food is and does can make mealtime a part of your training fun.

Mortal Dilemma: *I've heard that athletes need to eat a high-carbohydrate, low-fat, and low-protein diet. What changes must I make to my diet to be a successful long-distance athlete?*

Most people know the story of how "the Penguin's" running career began. In the event that you don't, I'll give you the short version. I was 43 years old and 240 pounds (80 more than today). I had smoked for 25 years and drank with the best of them. I didn't know the meaning of the word *nutrition*. My four food groups were sugar, caffeine, nicotine, and alcohol.

I had never before heard food defined as "fuel." Food as love? Got it. Food as comfort? Bring it on. Food as recreation? I understand. But food as something that my body actually has to use and convert to energy? No way.

—ᴍ—

As with John and so many others, food was anything but functional for me during my younger years. I had never thought of it as fuel for my body. I had always linked food with comfort. It wasn't until I visited a sports nutritionist that it all made sense. She asked me what, where, when, and why I ate. When I saw it all on paper, I realized I was running low on high-octane fuel.

Changing my eating behaviors was perhaps the most challenging part of training. My habits were so ingrained that I didn't even realize that I was reaching to food for help. One day at a time, I kept a journal and unwound the tangled mess of habits. Slowly, I began to create new eating behaviors and fuel myself optimally from the inside out.

Equating Food with Fuel

There are a lot of misconceptions about food and nutrition, and we hope to clear them up for you. This chapter will teach you when and how to fuel your body for optimal performance. We will discuss what to eat before, during, and after training and race day.

This subject is vast and entire books are dedicated to explaining optimal nutrition. If your interests are piqued and you find yourself wanting more, we suggest reading Liz Applegate's books and columns. She writes a monthly column for *Runner's World* and has authored several books on the subject.

Here's our take on the topic.

Food is a key ingredient to living a long and healthy life—something we need to move, to sleep, and to live. Food is to your body as gas is to your car engine. A car needs gasoline to function. If you fuel up with high-octane gas, your car will run efficiently. If you fuel up with cheap gas that has been watered down, it will put up a fight if it runs at all. If you don't regularly fill the tank with gas, you risk running out of gas and being stranded on the side of the road.

Our point is simple. You have the choice to fill your tank with high-octane fuel such as fruits and vegetables or risk lower-quality performance by fueling your tank with high-fat, high-sugar foods. It sounds simple, so why do we all struggle with food issues?

It bears repeating: Food is fuel. It provides the energy to get through your training as well as provides vitamins and nutrients to recover.

Calories In, Calories Out

Before we get into how to fuel yourself, we want to tell you a story about a girl named Jill. She joined a marathon training program for the sole purpose of losing weight. She thought that long-distance training would help her shed the extra 25 pounds she had been carrying around since her daughter was born.

Her training progressed, but she was shocked to learn she was gaining weight rather than losing it. She could not figure out why this was happening. After all, she was burning all those calories!

Here's what Jill was doing wrong. She was increasing her eating along with her mileage. She lived by the false assumption, "I just ran 12 miles, so I can eat whatever I want." Although at first, such thinking may seem logical, in the end it comes down to calories in versus calories out. Jill was consuming more calories than she was burning, and so she was ultimately gaining weight.

Training for a long-distance race is actually not the best time to plan on losing weight. You need to replenish your stores of carbohydrates, consume protein for muscle rebuilding, and depend on healthy fats to maintain your immune system. A healthy balance of all of these ingredients will keep your body running strong.

The Truth about Carbohydrates, Fat, and Protein

Carbohydrates are sugar. And despite popular belief, your body needs sugar.

Carbohydrates provide your muscles with quick "on the fly" energy fuel. Typically, we have enough carbohydrates stored in our muscles for 90 minutes of exercise.

Although your body always uses a ratio of carbohydrates, fats, and protein to function, it relies on a higher percentage of carbohydrates as you increase your exercise intensity. The faster or harder you go, the more sugars you burn. Carbohydrates serve as a quick but limited fuel source. They run out in a short period of time. Fifty to 60 percent of your diet should come from carbohydrates.

Let's move on to fat. Most people don't realize you need some fat to maintain a healthy immune system and nervous system. Eat too little fat and you risk lowering your immunity and getting sick. Eat too much fat and you risk gaining weight. Eat too much of the wrong *types* of fat and you risk clogging your arteries. Research indicates that your total caloric intake should consist of no more than 30 percent fat, with the bulk of it coming from healthy fat sources such as fish, flax, nuts, nut butters, avocado, and soy. Fat is not an enemy but rather an ally. In moderation, it will ward off illness and provide feelings of fullness or satiety.

Now for protein. It repairs and rebuilds muscle tissue. Research indicates long-distance athletes need a little more protein than the average person due to the stress of training and the constant muscle fatigue. On average 20 percent of your diet should consist of protein. This will aid in efficient recovery and restore your muscles for the next workout.

Low-fat, high-carbohydrate diet plans will only leave you spinning on a never-ending carbohydrate craving. Carbohydrates go through you quickly and, depending on what you eat along with them, cause your blood sugar levels to increase rapidly and then plummet, which makes you crave more carbohydrates. To avoid cravings and low blood sugar energy woes, eat frequently throughout the day with breakfast, lunch, and dinner and two snacks in between.

Mortal Miracle

"How has running made my life better? For the first time ever, I no longer have to try to survive on one lettuce leaf and one cup of coffee a day. I can eat *real food* (as long as I don't overeat), maintain a normal weight, and have better health than I ever had previously.

"Here's some background. I'm what horse people call 'an easy keeper.' It doesn't take much food to keep me going. So all my life I've had two alternatives: constant hunger or weight gain. Two years ago I weighed 60 pounds over normal weight for someone my size. I went on yet another diet. Finally, it hit me: In order to lose the weight and keep it off, I would have to exercise. I started walking. I started lifting weights, and the excess pounds came off faster!

"Seven months later I ran for 30 minutes for the first time ever in my life. Two months after that I ran my first 5-K race in 31:49 and won an age group prize. I was hooked."

—Pat, no age given

On the other side of that, low-carbohydrate, low-fat, and high-protein diets like the 40-30-30 plan can leave you lethargic during your training. Though the right balance is different for everyone, the general rule of thumb is to maintain a balance of 50 percent carbohydrates, 20 percent protein, and 30 percent fat. Try to balance of all these throughout the day, as they each play a vital role in digestion and metabolism. Consuming a pure carbohydrate meal such as pasta and red sauce or a pure protein meal such as steak and eggs will leave you out of balance and tired, hungry, or fatigued.

Starting Your Day Right

Breakfast is the most important meal of the day. This is the meal that "breaks" your fast from 8 hours of sleeping. It nutritionally "wakes" the body up. Most likely, if you struggle to keep your eyes open during the afternoon or come home to raid the cabinets, it is because you skip breakfast and your body is working on a low fuel tank. Just like your car, your body can run only if you fuel it properly.

Exactly how much and what you eat for breakfast depends on when you train.

If you don't train in the morning, eat your largest meal in the morning. Like a full tank of gas, it will keep you energized throughout the day.

However, if you do train in the morning, you'll follow a different strategy. You'll still eat breakfast, but not as much. You don't want to go without. Skipping breakfast and training in the morning is like heading for a long drive with a quarter tank of gas. You have just enough to get you there but nothing to get you back.

If you train in the morning, keep breakfast light and high in carbohydrates. A banana, half a Clif Bar, or a glass of juice will do the trick. Experiment with different foods and avoid anything high in fat or protein, as they take too long to digest and may cause stomach upset. Eat at least 1 to 2 hours prior to training. To pull this off, you may need to set your alarm at an ungodly early hour. Roll out of bed, eat your half a Clif Bar, take a short nap or complete some household tasks, and then head out for your run.

Because most races are held in the morning—likely including the one you're training for—experimenting with different breakfasts before a morning training session will help you determine what will sit well before your race. Practice, practice, practice. Your mission, if you choose to accept it, is to determine your prerace meal by experimenting with different types of meals before your morning sessions. To do this, you will need to try various foods. Come race day, you will realize it was time well spent.

Eating on the Run

Now comes the hard part. Remember when we said that your body eventually will run out of stored carbohydrates?

Well, for most people, that generally happens within 1 to $1\frac{1}{2}$ hours of running and walking. Because you will probably be on the roads for 2 to 8 hours for your half-marathon or marathon, you'll need to figure out what you can literally eat on the run. Again, practice is key. Experiment with different hydration and fueling strategies during your workouts. Come race day, you should have your fueling strategy firmly committed to memory.

When experimenting with fueling on the move, you must first determine the type of workout. Is it less than 60 minutes in duration or more than an hour in duration?

For Workouts That Last Less Than 1 Hour

Water is the key here. You're not walking or running long enough to exhaust your carbohydrate stores. However, you are out there long enough to sweat and breathe out a considerable amount of fluids.

Going without fluids risks dehydration, a condition that increases your chances for muscle cramping, a faster-than-optimal heart rate, headache, and fatigue. Consume 8 to 12 ounces of water every 15 minutes to avoid dehydration.

For Workouts That Last Longer Than 1 Hour

When John trains, he exercises for such long periods of time that he misses two entire meals while putting in his long miles. Although he recommends stopping at Starbucks to refuel, I've developed a different strategy.

Let's start with fluids. Like the shorter runs, you will need to fight off dehydration, especially in the warmer temperatures. Because we all have different sweat rates, some runners need more fluids than others. In general you want to consume 8 to 12 ounces every 15 minutes from the very beginning of your workout to the very end. If you are as forgetful as I am, set your watch timer to go off every 15 minutes to remind you to drink. It is the easiest way to avoid dehydration.

For these longer runs, you'll want to switch from hydrating with water to hydrating with sports drinks, a low-calorie mix of carbohydrates, water, salt, and potassium. Sports drinks are a must for fueling on long training runs and race day. They provide sodium, electrolytes, and energy in the form of fast-absorbing carbohydrates, all of which replenish quantities of sodium lost in sweat and sugar depleted from activity.

You'll find a plethora of drinks on the market and all have something to offer. Some drinks have been around forever, like Gatorade. Others, such as eFuel from CrankSports.com, are newcomers. This one in particular comes in a gel pack that you can easily dilute into water. It's a nice option for the marathon because you can add it to your water at each aid station, eliminating the need to carry heavy water bottles as you run.

To pick the best sports drink for you, decide whether you wish to train with the same drink that will be served on the racecourse. For example, if you know that the race is serving Gatorade at the aid stations, train with this drink to see how it sits with you. If your stomach revolts, then try other drinks—but know that you'll have to carry some with you on race day.

To solve this problem, invest in a water bottle pack. I've seen some marathoners wear fanny packs that even control the frequency and concentration of sports drinks.

Besides sports drinks, you can also consume other fuels that come in the form of puddinglike gel or sports bars. You can even choose other portable carbohydrate foods such as Gummy Bears, Twizzlers, and honey sticks. Experiment during your training runs, looking for a high-carbohydrate option that you can digest readily and actually enjoy eating.

Whether you consume gel or a bar, follow it with water to dilute it in your stomach. Also, avoid mixing gels and bars with sports drinks. The concentration of sugar will be too high and slow the absorption rate. So for calories on the run, either eat real food (a bar or gel) along with water *or* consume a sports drink. Don't combine the two.

Personally, I prefer gels. My favorite, eGel from CrankSports.com, tastes good, is easily digestible, and contains higher levels of electrolytes and antioxidants than most other gels. Gels offer a slight advantage over bars and hard food because they don't freeze in cold weather or melt in the heat. You don't have to chew. You just tear open the package and suck out the gel. If you can handle the taste, gels are the "on the fly" fuel of choice.

If you go with bars, choose bars that are low in fiber, protein, and fat. Any fuel other than carbohydrate digests slowly and may cause stomach upset. Stick with bars like PowerBar that contain high levels of carbohydrate.

Whether you choose a sports drink, gel, or bar, consume 50 to 100 calories every 30 to 40 minutes, or 100 to 200 calories every hour. If you're taller and weigh more, choose the higher calorie amounts. If you're short and skinny, go with the lower amounts.

Begin fueling 30 minutes into the session and continue throughout. If you wait until you feel hungry and tired, it's too late. Your tank will be empty and your car won't run. Fuel yourself frequently to maintain a steady flow of blood sugar, fluids, and electrolytes.

If you have a stomach of steel like John, you can start with a full concentration of sports drink, gel, or bar. If your stomach is highly sensitive like mine, try diluting the drink and gradually increasing the concentration over time. Try half a bar or gel at first and then graduate to a full bar. Your stomach will get used to the product, but it may take time.

One more tip: You want to get the fuel in you rather than on you. I spent the better part of a summer trying to master the drink-on-the-run technique. I never quite got it. I even went as far as carrying a straw with me to stick in the cups as I grabbed them.

I finally learned that simply stopping, walking, and drinking saved me more time than running and spilling. I made up the time later on the course.

Overloading Fluids

You're properly hydrated if your urine runs like lemonade or pale yellow. On average our bodies are up to 70 percent water. That includes our muscles, too! If you are low on fluids, your muscles are low on water and everything runs like a car very low on oil.

These days water is everywhere. It is "in" to drink water. There are even fitness waters like Propel that contain vitamins and minerals. They are low in calories but high in nutrients. Plus they are great tasting and easier to consume than plain old water.

Know that there is such a thing as overhydrating. In fact, a few long-distance runners, primarily women who walk or run-walk a marathon in over 4½ hours, have died from a condition called hyponatremia (low blood sodium).

We encountered this problem firsthand not long ago. We traveled to Dublin with 75 runners and walkers for a marathon and encouraged them to drink plenty of fluids to prepare for the race. One participant did just that, but she also made significant changes to her diet. She ate what she thought was healthy, sticking to mild, low-fat, low-sodium foods the week prior to the race.

On the 7-hour plane ride to Dublin, she drank 2 full liters of water and continued to do so until the race began two days later. Dublin is one of the few races that serves only water on the course, so she had no way of consuming a sodium-containing sports drink. As the race progressed, she depleted her sodium and potassium stores in her body. She continued to fuel her body with water, diluting the sodium in her blood. At the finish line, she had to be rushed to the hospital. We thought she was dehydrated, as the symptoms are similar: confusion, muscle weakness, nausea, and headache.

She came dangerously close to losing her life and was in a coma for well over a day.

That's the primary reason why plain water is not a good refueling tool for long-distance events. Instead, choose a sports drink that contains added sodium. Some experts even suggest that you eat a few pretzels or other salty snacks during the marathon.

Eating After the Event

You have a small window of opportunity postworkout in which your metabolism is revved up and, like a dry sponge, will absorb fuel readily and use it to replenish lost carbohydrates and electrolytes and rebuild your muscles.

In order for this to happen, you need to eat within the first 30 minutes of your longer workouts. If the thought of eating shortly after a workout isn't appealing to you, consume 200 to 300 calories of a sports drink or juice to tide you over until you cool down enough to develop an appetite. Within the next few hours, consume a balanced meal of about 400 calories that includes carbohydrates and protein.

The goal is to restock muscle glycogen with carbohydrates and repair muscle tissue tears with protein. Stay clear of high-fat meals, as they will slow the absorption and recovery rate.

Know Before You Go

The absolute most important nutritional step you can take to ensure marathon success: practice. As your longer workouts creep up in time and miles, begin experimenting with your pre- and postrun meals as well as your hydration and fueling strategies during your workouts. Experiment with different gels, bars, and sports drinks. Figure out the best way to carry your fuel on the run.

Remember:

- Food is fuel.
- Eating well is part of your training program.
- No diet is right for everyone.
- Long-distance training is not a weight loss program.
- You need more than water to be well-hydrated.
- Hydration is an everyday activity.
- Too much water is as dangerous as too little.
- Use sports drinks.
- Get the fluids in you, not on you.
- Eating after a hard workout speeds up recovery.
- Food is *fuel* that your body needs to perform.

CHAPTER TWELVE

Gear

Choosing the right equipment, from shoes and socks to sunglasses and hats, is just as important as choosing the right training plan.

Mortal Dilemma: *How will I know if I'm getting the right gear for me? What are the must-haves and what can I do without?*

—⚅—

People who know us know that we are both gear freaks who love to shop. Our shopping motto is "What's the worst thing that could happen?" If something looks cool, if something looks "trick," it goes into the shopping basket.

For example, one time we were passing through Fort Collins, Colorado, on the way to an expedition-length (7- to 10-day) adventure race in Idaho. We were reviewing our gear list and congratulating ourselves at having brought everything we could possibly need. Even so, we figured a short stop at the local outdoor store couldn't hurt.

Two hundred or so dollars later, we walked out carrying bags of gear we decided we simply *had* to have.

For the long-distance athlete, developing an interest and expertise in your equipment is secondary in importance only to your training. You need to learn about yourself, your feet, your body, your tendency to blister, your tolerance for heat and cold, your rate of perspiration, and so on in order to make wise decisions about the equipment you'll need.

You won't need all the gear it takes to do an expedition race, but you will need to make space in your closet for the clothes and shoes that you will need to get through training and the race.

In this chapter, we're going to start at the bottom, with your shoes and make our way up to your head. Dave and Lisa Zimmer, owners of Fleet Feet Sports in Chicago, are going to help us along the way. Dave will guide you in purchasing your shoes. And girls, Lisa is going to help you purchase the right "support system," or sports bra if you want to be technical.

Determining Your Arch Type

Before we get to shoes, though, let's take a look at your feet. We don't care if you have beautiful feet with well-manicured nails (like Jenny's) or the knarliest feet imaginable (like John's), the kind that look as if they were formed by a 3-year-old using Play-Doh. Whatever kind of feet you have, they are the ones that will carry you to the finish line.

We do care about the kind of arch you have. In general, a foot will have a high, normal, or low arch. High-arched feet are sometimes referred to as rigid feet; normal are referred to as—well—normal; and low-arched feet are sometimes referred to as flat feet. There are successful long-distance athletes with each of all of these kinds of feet. So whatever you have will work just fine. However, realizing what type of arch you have will help determine the best shoes for you.

The easiest way to decide what kind of arch you have is by doing the wet foot test. Soak the bottom of your foot and then step lightly on a piece of paper. A brown paper bag works best, but any paper will do in a crunch.

When you step lightly on the paper and remove your foot, you'll see a pattern. If you see a foot, chances are you have a normal foot. You'll see your heel, the ball of your foot, the outside edge of your foot, and your five toes (assuming you have five toes on each foot).

If you look down and see only your heel and the ball of your foot, you have a high-arched foot. If you look down and see a giant blob, you have a low arch.

A normal foot moves through the running and walking motion by striking on the outside of the heel, moving inward as your

Mortal Miracle

"I've run 12 marathons and 5 half-marathons. During those races, I learned that the two most important gear items are your shoes and a garbage bag.

"First, the garbage bag: You need it on race day, especially if it's cold or rainy. You can sit on it if you have to wait around before the event starts. And, you can dump it at little cost when you no longer need it during the race.

"Now for the shoes: I alternate training in two slightly different pairs and then purchase my favorite a few weeks before my event. I get about 30 to 40 miles in my new—but familiar—shoes before each marathon and always pack them in my carry-on when traveling."

—Philip, age 38

weight travels forward, and ending up on the ball of the foot as you push off at the end of the stride.

A high-arched foot moves through the running and walking motion by striking on the outside of the heel and staying on the outside of the foot. Even at the end of the stride, the high-arched foot tends not to move inward.

The low-arched or flat foot starts on the outside of the heel but then moves too quickly inward. What's worse is that as you travel through your running or walking motion, the low-arched foot doesn't stop moving inward. By the time you push off, you are almost standing on your ankles.

The movement of the foot from the outside edge to the inside edge is called pronation. Pronation is a good thing. You want to pronate. It's just that you want to pronate only as much as you need to.

A normal foot is said to have a neutral movement. A high-arched foot is likely not to move inward enough and is said to underpronate (or supinate if it actually moves outward), and a low-arched, flat foot will move inward too much and is said to overpronate.

Choosing the Right Kind of Shoe

Knowing what kind of arch you have is the first step in making a decision about a shoe. Shoes fall generally into a few large categories. An early caveat: Shoe companies don't agree which shoes belong in which categories. In fact, even their own brands add to the confusion. Don't worry about what a shoe is called or what category the manufacturer puts it in. Concern yourself only with your needs.

The most basic shoe is called a neutral shoe. This is, on the whole, the shoe on the lower end of the price scale and the one with the fewest bells and whistles. This doesn't mean it's a bad shoe. In fact, basic neutral shoes can be the best shoes for you. A higher price doesn't guarantee a better shoe.

The neutral shoes usually have midsoles that are all the same color. The midsole is just what it sounds like it is: that layer in between the upper part of the shoe and the sole which strikes the ground. Typically midsoles are white. If you have a neutral foot with a normal arch, it's quite possible that you can get away with wearing a very neutral shoe.

A word of caution: Never buy more shoe than you need!

Shoes with extra support on the medial (inside) of the midsole are called stability shoes. Probably 75 percent of all runners and walkers can get by with a decent pair of stability shoes. Again, just because one brand calls its shoe a stability shoe doesn't mean it is. It has to feel right.

Stability shoes usually have a two-colored midsole. The outer edge is usually white, and the inner edge, beginning at the heel or just inside the heel, is usually a deeper shade of gray. Different shoe companies use different materials, but the results are the same. They keep your foot from moving inward (or pronating) too much or too fast.

The most stable shoes are called motion control shoes. They are designed to control the inward motion of the foot as you go through the running or walking movement. In addition to the denser midsole material you'll find in the stability shoe, the motion control shoe will contain another feature to prevent your foot from rolling inward. This might be a plastic bridge at the arch or hunks of plastic in the inner heel. It doesn't matter. All the systems have the same goal.

The least stable shoes are called cushioned shoes. These shoes feel great in the store and when you take a few steps down the sidewalk. You'll feel like you've put pillows on your feet. It's tempting to believe that the cushioning is what you want and need. For nearly all of us, the highly cushioned shoe is an invitation to injury.

We'll explain. Whether your foot is normal, rigid, or flat, you still need some kind of relatively stable surface on which to run or walk. If you put a highly cushioned shoe below your foot, especially one that raises your foot inches off the ground, you have no stability at all.

Imagine strapping water balloons to the bottoms of your shoes. With each step the muscles around your joints react to the instability and try to keep your joints from going in every direction. The bottoms of your feet might feel good, but unless your biomechanics are perfect, take a pass on the cushioned shoes.

Finding the Right Shoe Size

Running and walking shoes shouldn't even have sizes on them. Not only do the manufacturers not agree among themselves as to what a size 9 is, they don't even agree within their own lines. So don't ask for the size that you've worn since high school and think it will fit. It won't.

You also can't buy a running shoe by its overall length. The critical measurement is not the overall length of the shoe, but the length of the arch—the distance between the heel and the ball of the foot.

Your running shoe has to fit your arch, not your foot. Some of us, like John, have long arches and short toes. This has resulted in his buying and wearing the wrong shoe size for nearly 5 years. The danger in having the wrong size is that the shoe won't bend at the same place your foot does, which, as you add on the miles, feels excruciatingly uncomfortable.

Shoe width is also something to consider. If, like John, you've got duck feet, you'll need to find shoes that are wide enough through the ball of the foot to accommodate your foot. You'll also need to consider the "volume" of your foot. If you've got a thick foot top to bottom, you'll need a shoe with enough room in the toebox to allow your foot to move without blistering.

There are enough high-quality shoes on the market that, with a little patience, you should be able to find a shoe that meets all of your needs. And when you do, that shoe will feel great from the first minute you put it on. If a salesperson tells you that the shoe will feel better once it "breaks in," leave the store. Modern shoes don't need to break in. Either they fit or they don't.

Put on the shoes and take them for a test drive. Walk around the store. Go for a little jog outside and pay attention to how they feel. Does your heel slide up and down? Do your toes feel cramped? Does any part of your foot slide or feel pinched against the shoe? A yes to any of those questions spells "no sale" for any pair of shoes.

Shoes, like tires on a car, wear out in time. The outsoles, the part that strikes the ground, lose their tread, the midsoles lose their cushioning and stability, and even the uppers (the part along the top of your foot) lose their shape and form. When? We can't say for sure. Even the best shoe won't last more than 6 months. At the first sign of a new ache or pain, blame your shoes and replace them immediately.

Adding Insoles and Orthotics

You can pay as much as $150 for a pair of shoes with the latest technology and still end up with a 15-cent insole or sock liner. Shoe companies seem unwilling to invest in quality insoles. Sure, there are a few exceptions, but on the whole, even great shoes contain lousy insoles.

Fortunately you can purchase a number of excellent options over-the-counter or through the trim-to-fit insole market. You'll find Superfeet and other brands at most running specialty and outdoor stores. These insoles can transform a very good shoe into the perfect shoe.

Despite popular belief, insoles are not the way to extend the life of a pair of shoes. The materials in the shoes are going to wear out regardless. Sticking a pair of soft insoles in a worn-out pair of shoes is a recipe for disaster.

Just beyond over-the-counter insole replacements, you'll find custom orthotics. These devices are made especially for you by a podiatrist. If you need orthotics, you need them. If you don't, they are a waste of money. In either case, we recommend that you exhaust all other solutions before you lay down the cash for custom orthotics, which can run you $200 or more and usually are not covered by insurance.

Socks

Let's start with the only absolute rule about socks: Cotton kills. That favorite pair of cotton tube socks that your kids gave you for your birthday might be fine for a casual softball game, but it will tear your feet to shreds in a long-distance training run or walk.

So buy synthetic. You've got plenty of options. Some people like thick socks. Brands like Thorlo and Smartwool, for example, make an entire line of socks that are well-padded at the heel and toe. Others of us like very thin socks. Brands like DeFeet and Patagonia make an excellent line of thin socks. Just keep in mind that the socks and the shoes have to match up. If you try on your shoes while wearing thin socks, you'll need to run in them wearing thin socks. Switching to thick socks will make your shoes fit too snugly.

Shorts and Tights

Let's start with the only absolute rule about chafing: Anything that rubs will chafe. John's battle with "chub rub" is well-documented. Even if he slathers on a layer of lubricant as thick as cake frosting, his thighs will create sparks before the end of the first mile.

This brings us to shorts. The two general categories of shorts are the traditional running short and the compression- or bike-style short. Deciding on which of these to wear is mostly a matter of personal preference, your level of modesty, and the aforementioned dreaded chafing.

The advantage to traditional running shorts is that they tend to be cooler than compression shorts and therefore more comfortable. Modern shorts contain a wicking brief and microfiber outer. Good shorts aren't cheap, but they are worth every penny if they keep you comfortable on your long training sessions.

The advantage of the compression shorts is that they will eliminate the chafing issue. They can also provide some measure of support for your hamstrings. They can also be, for some of us, not all that flattering. We're pretty sure that whoever invented Spandex didn't have hip, butt, and thigh issues. But these shorts do work.

The question that never gets answered because no one is willing to ask it is: What do you wear under the compression shorts? The answer isn't shocking. Some people wear nothing. Others wear some kind of brief. Do whatever makes you comfortable.

When to move from shorts to tights is also a very personal decision. It can be pretty cold outside before your legs will get cold during a long run or walk. More often than not, unless it is bitterly cold, you'll be better off in shorts. Our friend and colleague Eileen Portz Shovlin, the apparel editor at *Runner's World*, says she switches to tights only when the temperature drops below 40 degrees and opts for thicker, medium-weight tights when temperatures drop below 20.

Sports Bras

Today, there are almost too many bras from which to choose. To help you find the right bra for your needs, we called in the experts Lisa Zimmer, co-owner of Fleet Feet Chicago, and Sabra Bederka, Fleet Feet's operations manager. Here are their tips.

♦ Try on several styles and do a few exercises to see how each garment moves and feels. Doing jumping jacks or running in place works well.

♦ Look for breathable synthetic fabrics such as CoolMax that wick moisture away from the skin and offer a gentle supportive stretch that helps to minimize chafing.

♦ Stay away from cotton and any sports bra with a zipper. Although stylish, zipper bras score high on the chafing scale. They also can come unzipped.

♦ Wear the right type of sports bra for your bust size. There are basically two types of sports bras, the pullover type (a.k.a. the "uniboob") and the back-clasp type with individual cups.

Pullover bras usually work well for A- and B-cup runners. They can also work for women with larger cup sizes during lower-impact exercises such as walking or spinning.

Back-clasp sports bras generally come in C, D, and DD cups from 32 to 44. They also have adjustable shoulder straps to accommodate various cup sizes and volumes.

◆ Wear the right size. Surveys show that many women wear the wrong sports bra size. Use the following guide to measure yourself for the right sports bra size. Use a dressmaker's tape measure. Wear a regular lingerie bra that you think fits you well. Don't wear your sports bra.

1. Measure snugly around your rib cage, just underneath your breasts. Be sure the tape measure lays flat and even all the way around. You do not want the tape lower in the front or back.

2. Add 3 inches to your rib cage measurement. That equals your band measurement size. Measure around the fullest part of your bust, keeping the tape measure straight all the way around your body.

3. Subtract your band measurement from your breast measurement. This difference determines your cup size.

Difference	Cup Size
1"	A
2"	B
3"	C
4"	D
5"	DD

◆ Once you find the right sports bra, take proper care of it. Wash it on a gentle cycle and always hang it to dry. Machine drying breaks down the elasticity and support of the material.

Tops

You can break tops into three categories: singlets (sleeveless), short-sleeve, and long-sleeve. Like socks, the only rule is: Cotton kills. Your favorite T-shirt is not the perfect training shirt.

Each manufacturer has its own name for its technical fabric. It might be called Dri-Fit, Dri-Lete, or something like that, but it's just a fancy way of saying that it's a polyester-based fabric that is designed to wick the moisture away from your body. This wicking is important in hot *and* cold weather. In the hot weather you want the sweat away from your skin, out on the surface of the material where it can dry and cool you off. In the cold weather, you want the sweat away from your skin and moved to the outermost layer so that you'll stay warm and dry.

Your personal taste and modesty will dictate what kind of top makes you most comfortable. With the technical fabrics, there really isn't that much difference between a singlet and a short-sleeve shirt. The best option comes down to what you think you look and feel best wearing.

The decision to wear a long-sleeve technical shirt is a bit like the question about when to wear tights. It really comes down to your level of comfort and tolerance for cold. John tends to wear long-sleeve shirts in all kinds of weather because it's what makes him comfortable. The key is to experiment with your clothes during your training to eliminate the guesswork by race day.

Vests

One of the most important pieces of equipment for those of us who live in a three- or four-season environment is a running vest. You'd be amazed at how warm you can feel if you just keep the wind off your chest.

Your vest should fit snuggly enough to keep the wind out but not so tightly that it binds you. Since you will be wearing the vest directly over the base layer, you may find that it will be a size smaller than your jacket.

John's favorite vests are nothing more than a thin layer of nylon. However, newer vests are made of much more technical fabrics like Windstopper. Your budget, as much as anything, will help make that decision.

Fleece vests are great for layering under a shell for the morning hike in the woods, but they don't provide the warmth and protection you need for running. And unless you are running in extremely cold temperatures, a fleece vest with a shell will overheat you.

Some companies make running jackets with zip-off sleeves. These are jewels that are worth their weight in gold. If you don't already own one of these, buy it.

Hats and Headbands

Training through cold winters requires a hat or headband, depending on your body, the wind chill, and the temperature. In the coldest days of Chicago's brutal winter, most people wear a fleece or wicking hat to avoid losing precious heat through the head.

You can lose up to 40 percent of your body heat through your head. Without a hat, your body will have to shift gears to keep you warm rather than focus on moving you forward. There's also frostbite and wind chill to worry about.

Everyone has a different internal thermometer. Jenny puts on her headband when the temperature is 45 degrees and a fleece hat when it is 35 degrees. John is warm-blooded and wears a hat when it drops below 35. Hats keep you warmer and are geared to the colder temperatures, while headbands cover only your ears and work best in cool temperatures. If you live in a cold climate or will be racing in one, find out what your temperature gauge is and wear a hat or headband when needed.

The Cold-Weather Outfit Blues

Dressing for cold-weather workouts can be confusing. Our best advice: Dress in layers. That way, if you get overheated, you can shed a layer and keep moving.

The single biggest mistake made while training during the winter is overdressing. We remember the first cold day of our half-marathon training program. It was 40 degrees and everyone stood before us ready for a severe winter storm with hats, gloves, and big bulky jackets. Everyone had over-dressed, and within the first mile, layers were coming off and flying all over the path.

One easy way to determine whether you are overdressed it to use the "out-the-door" test. Dress so that you are chilled when you walk out the door for your workout. If you are warm before you begin, you will be too hot and risk overheating during the workout.

You don't need as much as you may think. Typically you should dress for 15 degrees warmer than the current temperature. That will account for your increased body temperature while moving and is a good gauge in deciding what to wear.

Heart Rate Monitors

There are more heart rate monitors than ever out there. You can choose from the most basic model that tells you nothing more than you are alive and your heart is beating. On the other hand, you can get one with all the bells and whistles, which will tell you your heart rate, your pace, your distance, and when you should call home to say hi.

Manufacturers like Polar, Nike, FitSense, CardioSport, and Timex make a variety of models from which to choose.

The right model and manufacturer is a very personal choice. If you are not interested in all the technical wizardry, then there's no sense spending all the extra money. If you like being distracted by an array of data, then there's no reason not to step up into one of the top-of-the-line models.

The Coolest Toy Since the Slinky

The first day I attached the Speed Distance Monitor from Nike to my running shoe, I felt like the girl in school with a brand-new bike. It instantly showed me my pace in minutes per mile, my speed in miles per hour, and how far I was running. What is better than that? It took over where the pedometer left off and removed all the guesswork in finding the right pace. I was immediately able to alter my pace and didn't have to drive the route to find out exactly how far I'd gone.

Speed Distance Monitors aren't required in training, but they are still valuable. I use mine all of the time to pace groups of walkers and runners. It teaches them to correlate the I-Rate system with speed and pace. They learn how they feel at different paces. It is cool and also useful—although, if you give me time, I can justify just about any toy.

Know Before You Go

If you haven't gotten to know the folks at your local specialty running store, take a field trip sometime soon. Bring in your running shoes and talk to the folks there about your marathoning plans and training. Tell them about any aches, pains, or discomfort along the way. Chances are that someone at the store will set you up with a piece of equipment that will make your training go so much easier.

Remember:

- Don't buy more shoe than you need.
- Don't buy shoes by their sizes.
- Pick a shoe based on the length of your arch, not your foot.
- Rotate your shoes.
- Even the best shoes wear out in about 6 months.
- Cotton kills.
- Quality running gear is worth the price.
- Never put your running gear in the dryer.
- It's your running gear, not an outfit; it doesn't have to match.
- When in doubt about the temperature, wear a little less than you need.

Part Four

Game Face

Getting to the starting line

takes more courage than finding

your way to the finish

CHAPTER THIRTEEN

Race Strategy, Goals, and Objectives

You can make the difference between having a great time and having the longest day of your life simply by developing your race strategy, thinking realistically about your goals, and planning carefully for your objectives.

Mortal Dilemma: *I understand why the people who are racing need to have a race strategy, but my only goal is to finish. Do I really need a strategy and objectives? Can't I just show up and see what happens?*

—⟋⟍—

Developing a race strategy does several things. First, it requires you to look honestly at your training and your overall readiness for the race. Second, it requires you to define your goals and look at them realistically. Third, it will give you something against which you can gauge your race as it's happening.

It also gives you something to do during the weeks when you are reducing your mileage and effort as you taper for your big event.

This is the time when your mileage is going down and your anxiety is going up. Suddenly you have hours in your life with nothing to do. You can take our word for it. You will want to find things to do during your taper just to keep you from going completely nuts.

First, let's start with your training. In developing a race strategy you have to look carefully at your actual training, not your fantasy training. Your body doesn't care about the miles you had *planned* to walk or run. It counts only the ones you put in. So when you look at your training log, look at only the miles you covered.

Go back and look at your initial goal, the one you wrote down way back in chapter 3. What was it then? Did it change as the training program progressed? Were you able to stay with your original goal, or did your life intervene?

How did you decide on that goal? Was it really your goal or had you, at the time, just adopted someone else's goal as your own? If you did adopt someone else's goal, now is the time to discard it and get your own.

How about the training? Did your training go exactly as you had planned? Were you able to commit the time, the days, and the miles that you said you could? Did the mileage add up more quickly than you thought it would? Were the long runs too long, too soon? Did you get in everything you had hoped to?

If not, it doesn't mean you're not ready; it just means that you're not ready for the race you had planned to run. And knowing that means that you can make the shift in your strategy now, before you line up, before you make a plan that is likely to lead to failure or frustration or injury.

How did the training affect you physically? Are you well-rested? Are you still working with a nagging injury of some kind? Are you sick to death of training and can't wait to get this over with? The truth is *your* truth. There are no right or wrong answers.

Based on your actual training, are you going to have to redefine your race goal? Do you think you overestimated or underestimated what the training program would do? Did you, at first, just want to finish, but now feel so great that you want to set a time goal? Did you have a time goal at first, but now would be happy just to see the finish line? The answers to those questions are important as you construct a race strategy.

There is nothing wrong with redefining your race goals now. Your chances of being successful are directly related to your ability to be honest with yourself. Only you know the answers that will lead to the best strategy.

Did you learn through the training program that long-distance running and walking is not an exact science? Did you learn on your long training days that no amount of planning can predict how you will feel on any given day? Did you learn that there are days when fast feels slow and slow feels awful? We hope so.

We hope you've learned that in spite of all the planning, nothing ever goes the way you think it will. We hope you've learned that you can't control any aspect of being a long-distance athlete except your willingness to participate in the process of preparation.

Race day is no different than any of your training days. Pinning a number to your chest doesn't guarantee an outstanding day or a record performance. Race day can feel magical. Race day can feel nightmarish. Most often, race day feels somewhere in between those extremes.

One Race, Three Plans

Despite all your introspection about your training, you still may need to change your race day strategy in the days or hours before the race—or even during the race. In fact, we recommend that you develop three race day strategies. Plan A, the "touched lightly by the race gods" strategy, would be one in which everything goes perfectly. In this strategy you sleep well the night before the race, you wake up feeling rested and refreshed, your breakfast settles well, and you are able to do all the things you need to do before you leave the hotel room.

The day is also perfect. It's overcast, about 45 degrees at the start, with no wind. You've brought exactly the right clothes. You remembered your favorite pair of shorts and top. Your socks are clean and soft. You tied your shoes just right the first time.

Mortal Miracle

"Soon after making a remarkable recovery from a river guiding accident that fractured my spine and pelvis, I moved to Washington state, took a desk job, got married, and became an instant mother. I stopped working out because of lack of time, and over the course of 4 years I gained 30 pounds. I didn't look fat, but I felt weak and heavy. I knew that I needed to do something right away.

"I set a 10-month goal to be in as good a shape by the time I turned 40 as I was when I ran track in high school. I started making time to work out again and added running to supplement my cardio.

"Soon, I started buying books on running, and decided that if I could run a marathon only 5 years after teaching myself how to walk again, then I could do anything. I finished that marathon. I can do anything!"

—Lisa, no age given

None of us gets very many of these days, but it's fun to think about them.

Plan B, the "most likely to happen" strategy, would be the one in which you show up with most of what you need and you manage to get in a few hours of restless sleep. You wake up grumpy. You barely manage to keep breakfast down, and your partner gets out of the bathroom only seconds before you threaten to kill him. Even then, your bowels decide to move 3 minutes after you leave the room.

The day is iffy. The forecast is for the chance of rain with the possibility of blistering sun or hail. It's 29 degrees at the start, but it's supposed to rise to the mid-90s by noon. You brought the pair of shorts with the worn-out elastic. You brought two mismatched socks. You've tied your shoes five times, and they still don't feel right.

For most of us, this is the way most race days feel. They aren't what you want them to be, but you can deal with what they are. Take our word for it—this is often as good as it gets.

Plan C, the "doomsday scenario" strategy (and yes, things could be worse than plan B), is the one in which the airline loses your luggage. You have to buy everything new at the race expo because you didn't pack all of your race gear in your carry-on bag. You didn't sleep a wink because there was a wedding reception in the room next door. You wake up feeling hungover, even though you didn't drink a drop. You can't even think about eating. Your partner decides she needs to soak in the tub for an hour even after you threaten to kill her. And your bowels decide to move 3 minutes after the gun goes off.

The day is miserable. It's either cold and damp or Death Valley hot and dry. The wind chill index is 60 degrees below zero or the heat index is 140 degrees. The race starts an hour and a half late.

The portable toilets are leftover from a motorcycle rally, and the guy next to you stomps on your foot as he yells "God bless America" at the playing of the national anthem.

Think it can't happen? It can. And it will happen to you at some point if you stay with the sport long enough.

—m—

My Penguin marathon strategy, for what it's worth, is one that I've developed carefully over the past 10 years. I've modified it some as I run more marathons. Now that I've run more than 30 marathons, I think I've got it refined to the point that I'm willing to share it with you. Here goes.

The Penguin Marathon Strategy: Finish the same day that I start.

Okay, there's some humor in that strategy, but it's as good a place to start as any. If you're a first-timer, you can't even begin to develop a strategy based on anything other than pure speculation and wild guessing. You might believe that you can look at some of your longer runs and make some predictions based on those times, but it doesn't always work that way.

Long-distance races are mysteries. I like to think of them as theater, plays in which I have my part, but I'm not given a script. I'm given my lines 1 mile at a time. Every new mile marker offers a place to take my role in some new direction.

Goals

Having a strategy is not the same as having goals. Goals are things that can be met or not met. Goals are lines or points on the map that will tell you how far you've come or how far you've gone. And while goals can be met, they can also be missed.

To develop your goals, you first must understand the volume of the distance; 13.1 or 26.2 miles are a *long* way. Most new long-distance runners line up thinking that their goal is to run or walk 13.1 or 26.2 miles. That's all well and good at the start.

As the race goes on, however, you'll find that your goals keep changing. If you're in a marathon, you may find yourself thinking in smaller chunks of distance. Your goal might be to get to the 5-mile mark or the halfway point. For some of us, in the later stages, the goal changes to getting to the next mile marker or the next tree. In the end, for all of us, our goal becomes just taking that last step across the finish line.

One of my adventure-racing buddies once asked me, in the middle of an overwhelming 60-mile jungle trek, "Jenny, how do you eat an elephant?" When I winced at the thought of thinking about anything but my sore feet, he replied, "One bite at a time."

I still use that little bit of knowledge whenever I see a nervous walker or runner at the starting line of a long race. It is true: If you think about completing the whole distance in one bite, it seems impossible. But if you break the distance down into bite-size pieces, it doesn't sound so bad.

You can do this in miles or by geographical landmarks. Identify several landmarks to find scattered on the course. The race becomes a mental scavenger hunt for the landmarks. Another trick is to pick specific mile markers balanced throughout the course, such as mile 3, 6, 9 and the finish line. It doesn't matter how you choose to divide it as long as you do. Then you end up crossing several mini–finish lines rather than just one big one.

—◊◊—

Goal setting is a tricky business even for the very best competitors. I, John, get very upset when I see first-time long-distance athletes finish with their heads hanging down. I see them at the finish line and they look like they just lost their best friends. Even as the volunteer hangs the medal around their neck, they look disappointed.

When I ask them why they're disappointed, the answer is almost always the same: They had a goal to finish in a certain time and they missed it. When pressed for how they came up with the goal that they missed, it's almost always based on voodoo science. And it nearly always failed to take into account the course, the day, and their states of mind.

Sadly, their disappointment is often a result of their inexperience as well as an incomplete understanding of the difficulties and vagaries of long-distance racing. The more experience you have, the more likely you will take the race as it comes and will be prepared to change your goals at a minute's notice.

Objectives

Objectives are not exactly the same as goals. Do you know the metaphor about the alligators and the swamp? When you're up to your butt in alligators, it's hard to remember that your objective was to clear the swamp. The same is true for long-distance races. When you're up to your butt in the realities of the race, it's hard to remember that your objective was to finish strong and unassisted.

An example of an objective would be to stay hydrated. How you accomplish this objective isn't a given, and unlike a goal, you have to plan for and prepare for your objectives. It's never enough just to have an objective. You have to think carefully through the processes and procedures necessary to implement the objective.

Let's take the hydration example. You've done your homework. You know that the Mule Barn Marathon will have fluid stations at every mile. Each station will have both water and a sports drink. You've trained with the sports drink, you know how much you can tolerate, and you're ready to meet your objective.

To meet that objective you might plan to take water at every fluid station and sports drink at every other. That all sounds good. In most cases, if a race advertises that there will be water and sports drinks at every mile, they will do everything in their power to make sure it happens. But . . . things happen.

Race organizers make predictions on how much water and sports drink to have available at each station. An unusually hot day, or some other unforeseen circumstance, could mean that their predictions are off by 10, maybe 20 percent or more. If you happen to be in the last 20 percent of the field, you may find that you are SOL—Short Of Liquid.

All of a sudden, your objective of staying hydrated has gone right out the window, and so has your race goal and race strategy. Most important, in this case, not planning for such an unpredicted contingency can put you in real danger.

So, it's not enough to pick "to stay hydrated" as one of your objectives and think you're finished. You've got to take time to think about how and where you'll meet that objective, what you'll do if your first plan doesn't pan out, and how you'll handle the best-case, worst-case, and doomsday scenarios.

Another common objective is to stay well-fueled during the race. These days that almost always means carrying those ubiquitous foil packets filled with gel. Again, assuming that you've done your homework, practiced what kind and how many gels you'll need and when, and decided how you'll carry enough with you, it sounds like you'll just line up and be fine.

Not so fast there, Red Rider. What happens if this isn't your best day? What happens if you end up on the course 30 minutes or an hour longer than you had planned? What then? Well, if you're not prepared, the race will go from bad to worse in a hurry.

—ɯ—

This has happened to me, the Penguin. In fact, it has happened to me more than once. I had great objectives, solid planning, and lousy execution. Am I particularly stupid? I don't think so. It's just that things happen in long-distance races that you can't predict. Being prepared for anything is the only objective that will work.

One example seems worth detailing. I was asked to "pace" a marathon at the last "official finish" pace for Team in Training at the Mayor's Midnight Sun Marathon in Anchorage, Alaska. I had to finish in 8½ hours. The pace was too slow to run and just a little too fast to walk comfortably. I was sure that after 32 marathons, I could just figure it out as I went along. Wrong. Run/walking 32 marathons in the 5- to 6-hour range doesn't tell you a thing about walking a marathon in 8½ hours.

I had no idea how to space out my hydration over that length of time. I had no idea how to space out my food intake, my gel intake, and the inevitable onset of fatigue. The result was one of the ugliest last few miles of a marathon that I have ever suffered through.

Poor planning? Yes. Failure of imagination? Yes. Inability to predict the future based on the past? You bet. It can happen to any of us at any time no matter how well-prepared or experienced we are.

—∿∿—

The pace at which you begin the race will quickly determine the outcome of your journey. Sounds profound, doesn't it? It is. Like John, I learned this the hard way. Also like John, some of my greatest lessons have been the result of adversity.

It was a crisp morning in Milwaukee. I signed up to run the Lakefront Marathon with the lofty goal of qualifying for the Boston Marathon. I knew I was in trouble when I looked down and my shorts didn't match my top.

I had trained hard and rested well. My body knew the exact pace to the second that I needed to qualify for Boston. I had to run even miles at an 8:20 pace. Imagine my surprise when I hit the first mile in 7 minutes flat! Now, you may think that being a minute and 20 seconds ahead of pace at mile 1 would be a good thing, but it isn't. It's the worst mistake you can make. (I'll explain in a bit.) If that wasn't bad enough, I ran right by the first fluid station because there were so many people there and I didn't want to waste any time.

By mile 10 I was cussing out the squirrels, and by mile 18 I was crawling. I couldn't see. I couldn't count to 10. To make matters worse, I was crying.

What was I thinking? That's the point. My body showed up on race day rested and ready to go. My training had gone like clockwork. Every mile was productive and every rest day restful. Unfortunately, showing up on race day well-trained isn't the last step.

In order to complete the distance successfully, your mind and body must work in unison. I had to drop out of the race because my nerves encouraged my mind to take my body hostage. I made every mistake in the book.

The best long-distance athletes aren't necessarily the fastest. The most successful athletes use their smarts to guide their bodies through strong races. Make your goal to conserve energy in the first half of the race so that you can finish strong at the end. We refer to this as negative splits, and it's harder than it sounds. If you don't believe us, watch the end of a long-distance race. There are people limping, crawling, and sometimes swaying in the last few miles— all because they went out too fast.

If you play your cards right and stay with your pace strategy from the very beginning, you will pass the "swaying athletes" en route to a strong finish. This takes patience and discipline. Once the gun goes off and the horses leave the gate, it's a free-for-all. The horses that finish strong keep their own paces and stay true to their pacing strategies. Take it out slow, conserve your energy, and finish the second half strong.

How do you learn pace? I'm glad you asked. One of the greatest ways to learn pacing strategy is to run a few 10-K races. Use the race to experience the prerace jitters, the adrenaline rush of the crowd, the art of drinking fluids during a race, and, most important, staying with your pace strategy no matter what is going on around you.

Another way to learn to stay with your pace strategy is to invest in a Speed Distance Monitor. If you struggle with learning to pace yourself, this training tool will do the trick. It instantaneously reads your pace in minutes per mile and miles per hour *and* gives you your mileage. It's like moving on a treadmill with all the numbers right there in front of you.

Going with the Flow

Your greatest danger is not the course or the distance. Your greatest danger may be your unwillingness both to accept the difficulty of the challenge before you and, as a result, to refuse to adjust your strategy, goals, objectives, and even your definition of success.

There is no right strategy. There is only *your* strategy. But—and this we believe with all our hearts—it is important to develop some kind of strategy. We don't want to see all of your hard work and training fall apart because you failed to have a strategy, or failed to set realistic goals, or—worse—didn't think your objectives through very carefully.

If you are prepared to spend months training, we think it's well worth the time it takes to spend a few hours developing your race strategy, your race goals, and your personal objectives. The time you've spent training your body is already in the bank. Now you can apply your intellect to help you achieve your maximum performance.

Know Before You Go

Take a moment to think about your race day strategy. How will you motivate yourself when the running gets tough? What pace will you run? How will you carry food and how often will you eat it? Have you practiced your race day strategy during training?

Remember:

- Your goals, strategy, and objectives have to work together.
- Penguin race strategy: Finish the same day you start.
- Be prepared to change your goals on race day.
- Be prepared to change your goals as the race unfolds.

- Keep your objectives firmly in your mind.
- If you can't be well-prepared, be well-rested.
- There is no such thing as the perfect race.
- Imagining a race is not the same as running or walking it.
- A bad strategy is worse than no strategy.
- Relying on race day magic is like believing in Santa Claus.

CHAPTER FOURTEEN

Race Preparation

After months of training, the big day is finally here. The planning is over, the training is over, and the tapering is over. You've got your plan and your strategy. It's time to roll.

Mortal Dilemma: *Okay, you two,*
I've done everything you said to do. I've trained smart.
I've put in the time and the miles. I've tapered well.
How do I make sure that I've done everything I need to do
in order to have a successful race?

This is where the real fun begins. Those last few days and hours before the big event are filled with excitement, terror, joy, frustration, calm, and panic. It's the best time of all.

At least it can be the best time of all. It can be if you're open to the mood of the moment and the sometimes wild swings of emotions from well-placed confidence to abject terror. If this is your first time, the last few days before the goal event will be unlike anything you've ever experienced. The emotions feel like a cross between a surprise birthday party and jumping from the 100th floor of a building.

Here's your first rule for race prep: Understand that whatever you're feeling is normal. If you find yourself waking up in the middle of the night screaming—that's normal. If you find yourself singing every Grateful Dead song you ever heard—that's normal. And if you find yourself suddenly living in a parallel universe where no one else seems to understand a word that you're saying—that's normal, too.

Don't worry if your friends and family don't understand you. Don't worry if by the Thursday before race day no one is even willing to be in the same room with you, let alone try to have a conversation with you. These last few days are the closest to being possessed that you will ever experience. Rather than fighting it, enjoy it.

We'd like to be there for this marvelous journey. To do so, we'll start with what you will experience and what you should do from 3 weeks before the big day, counting down to toeing the start line. Let's go.

3 Weeks Before the Big Day

You'll dedicate the last 3 weeks of your training program to recovery and rejuvenation. We refer to this as tapering. The volume of mileage decreases gradually, allowing your body to recover from the demands of progressive training. Although you may want to train harder during these weeks, that tactic will only hurt your performance.

It's a well-documented scientific fact that long-distance athletes suffer from Taper Madness in the last few days before the goal race.

The symptoms of Taper Madness are also well-documented. They include but are not limited to:

1. An unnatural need to spend money
2. An attraction to buying hideous running apparel
3. A "must-have" mentality toward running toys
4. A complete aversion to running

Three weeks before a goal race marks an extremely dangerous time. While Jenny somehow is able to exert a little more self-control, if I'm not careful, I'll buy a new car, a piece of retirement property, and a gravesite during the last 3 weeks. Even though I've been through it before, it still catches me by surprise. How else do I explain the pair of leopard-skin tights that are in the bottom of my drawer of running clothes?

Mortal Miracle

"I started running with a guy I was dating. We would run together almost every day, with him constantly telling me that I was not as fast as he was, etc. The relationship ended about a week before the race we were training for. I was determined to beat him and had quite a good finishing time. I saw him a week or so after and learned that he had slept in and didn't run. His comment told me two things. One, I was smart to end the relationship. Two, I was addicted to running. I have since run 4 marathons (including Boston) and about 10 half-marathons. My husband is not a runner, but he understands my commitment and is totally supportive."

–Jill, age 38

And running toys? The sillier and the more ridiculous, the more likely I will buy it during Taper Madness. A waist belt that contains a water bottle carrier and a pocket for a cell phone? Got to have it. A wristwatch, heart rate monitor, GPS, digital camera? Absolute must-haves on race weekend.

I'm convinced that the only reason the big events have expos on race weekend is because organizers know that the participants will spend massive amounts of money on stuff they don't need and won't use. How else do I explain my 17 pairs of cotton gloves?

Fortunately I've discovered a method for easing the Taper Madness and related prerace jitters. Here goes: Distill your running life down to the things you can see and feel. Find all the things that you can touch. Gather up all the running shoes and socks and clothes that you own and put them in a bag. Wrap yourself in T-shirts and jackets that make you feel good.

The last 3 weeks before a race, I try to wear only clothes that make me feel good. This is not the time to try to squeeze into a pair of slacks that you haven't been able to wear since high school. This is also not the time to shop for new clothes. Your body has been making the adjustments necessary to run a long-distance race, not to go to a 10-year high school reunion.

I usually take all the running clothes in my closet, launder them, and put them in a giant bag. I do this because I'm certain that if I forget one piece of running apparel, one sock, one singlet . . . then, on race morning, I'll decide I need that exact piece of apparel. So I'm not taking any chances.

It doesn't matter what time of year it is or where I'm racing; I'm still going to take at least one of everything I own. This thoroughness (some might say obsession) is born of experience. I've run in freakishly hot weather in the middle of winter and in freezing rain on the 4th of July. I've seen it all, and I'm sure that I'll see it again. So my advice is: Take it all.

1 Week and Counting

During the week before race day, start paying close attention to what you're eating. We hope, of course, that you've learned during your training what works and what doesn't in your system. The week before the race is no time to start experimenting with "Foods from Around the World." Stay with what you know.

If you've been eating well and properly during your training, you shouldn't have to make any changes. You should hopefully have already learned that a greasy burger and fries aren't the best prerun meal. Even so, in the last few days, monitor your food intake with even more rigor. You may find that even some of your favorites don't sound good during this time.

If you, like we do, sometimes turn to food for comfort, this last week can mark a dangerous transition for you. You may find yourself reaching for food to help ease your anxiety or to help pass the time. Be careful, but don't beat yourself up if you slip a time or two. In the week before the big event, you will probably crave comfort foods. It's okay. Eat what makes you feel good. You are not going to gain enough weight in a week to make that much of a difference.

If you develop a nervous stomach prior to the race, try eating smaller amounts of food more often. Even then, focus on foods that are easy to digest.

Race week is *not* the time to try to diet. Because you've backed off from your high-mileage training weeks, your appetite may be a little off-kilter. That's normal. You may be hungrier than you've been. You may not want to eat anything. Whatever you're feeling, try to maintain the best eating habits you can.

Staying well-hydrated during that final week is also critical. This doesn't mean you must strap a 50-gallon drum of water to your back, but it does mean you should be more aware than ever of the amount of water that you're drinking—and not just water. Make sure that you're taking in the electrolytes (sodium and potassium in particular) that you'll need on race day. Sipping sports drinks is a great way to keep your electrolyte stores filled to capacity.

The Night Before

Despite popular belief, you don't need to "carbo-load" the night before the race. The whole concept of carbo-loading is a throwback to the dark ages of long-distance running. We still like to have pasta parties the night before a race, but they've become more social and psychological than physical.

In the good old days, long-distance runners would go out and run about two-thirds of the race distance—and run it hard—about a week before the event. The idea was to run all of the glycogen (or carbohydrates) out of their systems. They would intentionally deplete their systems of the glycogen they needed to run. Make sense? Not really.

Then, early in race week, these old-timers would eat almost nothing but protein—avoiding carbohydrates altogether—just to make sure that they had no glycogen at all stored in their livers and muscles. This carbo-depletion also had the side benefit of pulling lots of water weight off their bodies so that they had the impression of being lean and mean.

On the night before the big race, they would carbo-load to try to replace the liver glycogen. They would do this by eating plate after plate of pasta or rice. This, of course, did put the carbs back in their system but also caused them to bloat up like crazy because of water retention.

It's a wonder these folks could run at all. It also explains why this form of carbo-loading led to some very nasty-looking carbo-unloading sometime during the race.

The general balance of your diet needn't change as race day approaches. The day before the event, you may want to stay away from foods that you know are hard for you to digest. Twelve hours before the race isn't the best time to eat a huge chicken Caesar salad! And Saturday night before a Sunday marathon is not the time to try 10 different levels of curry at your favorite Indian restaurant.

Those Last Dreadful Hours

Once you are back your hotel room, counting down the hours until race start, it's time to think seriously about your race wardrobe. Since you've brought every piece of running apparel you own, this shouldn't be a problem.

Even after 30-plus marathons, I still lay out, and put on, exactly what I think I'm going to wear on race morning. I'm not talking about looking into my luggage and making sure it's all there. I'm talking about taking it all out, putting it all on, taking it all off again, and laying it out in reverse order—fireman style.

This is the point where I completely obsess about my number. I know just where I want it to be. I know that it has to be pinned on in just such a way that it hangs down over my waist. I don't want it up too high or it will make my stomach look big. I don't want it too low or it will make my legs look short. I'm not kidding!

Mortal Miracle

"I was a procrastinator and a quitter for much of my life. I was a lousy paperboy when I was 13. I waited to turn in mediocre papers until the last minute in high school. I dropped out of college in 1982.

"Then, when I began to run and then decided to tackle a marathon, my life and attitude began to change. I designed a training schedule and stuck with it. I began to believe in the value of self-discipline and goal setting.

"I realized I could apply the same type of mental and physical effort to studying or working. I finally finished my undergraduate degree and have earned a master's degree. I went on to run four more marathons."

—Steven Friedman, age 43

If this is your first long-distance event, it's worth whatever time it takes to get that number exactly where you want it. You know you're going to want to buy the finish line photo and you are not going to want to look at a crooked number for the rest of your life.

With the proliferation of sports drinks, bars, and gels (and other energy and electrolyte replacement products coming soon), it is also a good idea to do some calculations on what you think you'll want to bring with you for the race. The general rule of thumb on the energy gels, for example, is that you'll need to suck down one about every hour. If you're planning to finish in about 5 hours, then you'll need to find a way to carry 4 gels. There are lots of ways to carry gel, from pinning the packets to your shorts to wearing a belt with bottles filled with the stuff. How you carry it doesn't matter, but deciding on how to, and how much, is something you need to do before race morning.

You don't need to worry about having the time to do all this. You'll have more than enough time because you are not going to sleep much. You're not. So just forget about it. You may try to sleep. You may lie in bed and toss and turn for hours. But you're not going to sleep.

On big race days, I set three alarms—three separate alarms. I have a travel alarm and two different watches. If it's a critical race with an extremely early start, I'll even order a wake-up call from the front desk. Even with that, I've never been asleep when any of the alarms went off!

Race Day

If you do fall asleep, make sure to get up when you wake up. Even if that's well ahead of when you wanted to get up, it's better than staying in bed and just waiting. There's always something you can do, so get up and get going.

I, John, will often throw on some clothes and go outside early in the morning. It doesn't matter to me that the race doesn't start for another 4 hours; I want to see the weather for myself. I pretend I actually know what it means if the sky is clear or cloudy. I repeat the old sailing adage—Red sky at night, sailor's delight; red sky at morning, sailor take warning—even though I don't have the faintest idea what the red sky indicates.

Mostly, I just want to get out of the room and get moving around. It doesn't matter if I don't know what I'm doing; at least I'm doing something.

Breakfast on race day is something worth thinking about. My best advice is to eat what you normally eat for breakfast (or what you discovered worked for breakfast on your long training runs) but eat only about half as much. It's not unusual to have butterflies before a big race, so eating a little less than normal is a pretty good plan.

Even as I write this, I know that there are great runners who will load up on eggs, sausage, and gravy and still go out and have a fantastic race. There have even been times when I've been willing to tempt fate and eat a less-than-ideal breakfast, but it's not a good idea. Eat what works. Just don't eat too much of it.

It's always important to get to the race start site early. It's especially important at a big race. And this next sentence is the most important sentence in the entire book: When you get to the race site, *immediately* get into a portable-toilet line. I'm not kidding. Do not stop to talk. Do not look around for friends. Make a direct line for the portable toilets.

I don't care how often you go to the bathroom before you leave the hotel; you are going to need to go again before the race starts. Don't take any chances. Get in line.

When you've gotten to the front of the line, then gotten in and out of the portable toilet, get back in line again. Trust me on this one. Stay in the portable toilet line until you have to line up for the race.

Making sure that you line up in the right place is important to you and your fellow competitors. Nothing can spoil a race for a new racer and the experienced racers like lining up too far forward in the pack.

Many races have projected mile times up on signs or have the participants grouped into "corrals." Whatever the organizing scheme, you want to make sure that you are in the place you need to be. Once the gun goes off, you do not want to find yourself surrounded by hordes of participants who are going out at a pace faster or slower than you.

If the race organizers don't give any indication of where you should stand, then it's up to you to find out where you belong. The easiest way to do this is to ask. Honest. Just ask the person next to you what time they hope to finish in. If you're hoping for a 5-hour marathon and the person next to you is hoping for a 3:30 marathon, one of you is in the wrong place. If you're new to the sport, assume it's you.

It's just as important not to line up too far back. Don't be overly modest about your goals. Be honest. If you have prepared for and are capable of running a 9-minute pace for this event, then you have every right to line up with the other 9-minute milers, regardless of whether this is your first race.

Once you're in the pack where you belong, there's not much left to do but wait for the start. I try to use these last few minutes to do a final check on everything from my shoes to my hat. Once I'm out there on the course, it's too late.

Besides, if you've gotten this far, if you are standing in the pack at the start of your goal race, you have already accomplished more than most. Take the time right there and then to congratulate yourself.

For you, and for the hundreds or thousands of other participants, the party is just about to begin.

Know Before You Go

You've put in the training. You're ready to go the distance. You're normal. Just do it. Aim to finish the same day that you start, and you'll do just fine. We're proud of you. See you after the race!

Remember:

- Don't try anything new on race day.
- Don't try *anything* new on race day.
- Whatever you are feeling during race week, it's normal.
- Don't try *anything* new on race day.
- Pay even more attention to what you eat the week before the race.
- Don't try *anything* new on race day.
- Staying hydrated all week is as important as hydrating during the race.
- Don't try *anything* new on race day.
- *Don't try anything new on race day.*

CHAPTER FIFTEEN

It's All About the Medal

In the largest events, nearly 40,000 runners, run/walkers, and walkers start with hearts filled with hope and desire. Somewhere in front of them are a finish line and a medal. For most, those are all the reward they need.

Mortal Dilemma: *It's the night before the race and I'm starting to wonder what the heck I was thinking when I decided to do this. Can you please remind me?*

As I, John, sit here tapping the keys of the laptop, thinking about telling you about my first marathon finish, I can feel the hair on my arms start to stand up. It's been nearly a decade since I crossed that first marathon finish line, but I can remember the feeling like it happened just a few hours ago.

I told you earlier that it took me nearly 10 months to finish that first marathon—not because I'm *that* slow, but because I did such a terrible job of training for the first attempt that it took that long to recover and train for my second attempt with a little more common sense. The time between the first starting line and first finish line probably made the accomplishment even more special.

The place was Columbus, Ohio, in the fall of 1993. The day, I can tell you, was perfect—cool but not cold, sunny but not too bright. The crowd, the course, and the conditions all conspired to make this the day of a lifetime. Ten years and 30 marathons later, I've still never had a better day. And I mean that in every sense of the word.

I lined up next to my friend Lee. He was, at the time, the only person that I actually knew who had completed a marathon. In fact, even back then he had completed something like 70 marathons. He was my coach, my mentor, my hero, and my best friend on that day. Together, every step of the way, we ran and walked and talked our way through a simply glorious day.

For some reason, I decided to wear a train engineer's hat. Even now, I can't tell you why. I might have been thinking about "the little engine that could." I really don't know. Keep in mind that this was years before people started calling me "the Penguin," so it wasn't like I was trying to create an image.

I also wore a cotton, long-sleeve biking jersey. You read that right. A red, cotton, long-sleeve biking jersey. The kind with pockets across the back. I filled those pockets with energy bars and ibuprofen, which, at the time, I thought was all you really needed to finish a marathon.

To complete the outfit, I chose a pair of latex compression shorts. I have always believed that anything that can chafe will chafe, and I was forever dealing with a major-league case of "chub rub." I was, to say the least, a sight.

A 45-year-old man in an engineer hat, red cotton biking jersey, and black compression shorts. Think about it.

Before that race, my longest run ever had been 15 miles. That seemed like plenty. I had been so overtrained for the first attempt that I figured this time I was taking no chances. It's better, I thought, to be a bit undertrained than overtrained. As it turned out, it wasn't such a bad idea.

I planned to use a modified Jeff Galloway run/walk program. (Jeff Galloway, a former Olympian, pioneered run/walking. At the time, it was a controversial and completely new technique for completing a marathon.) Lee and I were going to run for 20 minutes and walk for 2 minutes. I can't remember now why we decided on that particular interval. Most likely it was just something that came to us in a vision. Whatever the reason, that was our plan and we stuck with it.

The day went about as well as it could, right up to the infamous mile 20. Mile 20 is "the Wall." For many runners and walkers, this is where the marathon starts. As a friend of mine used to say, the marathon is 20 miles of hope followed by 6 miles of truth. I know that's where everyone says the Wall is, but this wasn't like hitting a wall. This was like someone handing me a refrigerator and asking me to carry it to the finish line. It wasn't that anything hurt. It was as if I suddenly weighed 800 pounds.

But I pressed on because I didn't know any better. I pressed on because I knew there was a finish line out there somewhere. I pressed on because, at the time, the idea of not pressing on didn't occur to me.

Then suddenly (after nearly 5 hours) there it was: the finish line. The crowd had thinned to just a few die-hard volunteers and a few goodhearted friends and family of those of us who were leading the end-of-race ambulance like a small band of wounded soldiers. But the finish line was there, the same line that the winner had crossed more than 2½ hours earlier.

Mortal Miracle

"Since childhood, I have marveled at athletes in many sports and dreamed of an Olympic gold medal or a Heisman trophy. Unfortunately, I was blessed with only average athletic ability and made only modest achievements in high school middle-distance running. I've now run three marathons and am training for my fourth. I'm on the verge of qualifying for Boston. I have achieved the glory as an athlete that I have sought my entire life!"

—Chris, age 31

In a single step, my life changed forever. In 4 hours, 57 minutes, and 32 seconds, I had undone a lifetime of not finishing. In just a little less than 5 hours, I had erased 45 years of failure. With that one step across the finish line, I became something I never dreamed I could become. I became an athlete.

Even better was that I became an athlete with a medal. A medal. For me, it couldn't have been more exciting if it had been an Olympic gold medal. It was a medal. It was a medal that someone hung around my neck. It was a medal that I could keep, that I could show people, that I could brag about, and that I could use as a reminder that for at least 1 day in my life I had succeeded.

One Small But Significant Step

In the years since that day, I've crossed more than 30 more marathon finish lines and seen tens of thousands of runners and walkers cross finish lines all over the world. One thing stands out:

Something very personal and very deep happens somewhere between the last step and the medal.

I've seen participants come across the finish line crying like babies. Their eyes are so filled with tears that I wonder how they can see to run or walk. Once in a while I've gone over and hugged those folks because it seemed like the only thing I could do.

One young man in particular stands out. He was in his mid-twenties. There wasn't anything all that unusual about him. He was, or so it seemed, just one of hundreds of young men out there in Austin, Texas, on that February morning. He wasn't fast, he wasn't gifted, and he wasn't special in any other way. Yet that young man has become a memory seared into my brain.

As he crossed the finish line, he began to cry—not just the "filled with emotions from finishing" kind of crying, but a gut-wrenching, blood-curdling wail that was coming from some part of him that had been liberated by the distance and the effort and the step across the finish line.

He was nearly my son's age, so I did what I supposed was the "fatherly" thing and just ran up and hugged him. Actually, I just stood there and held him for fear that his emotions would carry him away. I don't know how long we stood there locked in the embrace, but it was long enough that my arms were getting tired.

Then, as suddenly as it started, it ended. He released his grip on me, wiped the tears from his eyes, thanked me, and walked away. I didn't know who he was then, and I don't know who he is now, but I can tell you that I do know I shared in a moment of release unlike any other I have ever experienced.

Oh, the young man's time? Just over 5 hours. Five hours.

Would that experience have been any different for him if had finished in 3 hours? Given his modest physical talent, could he have ever had that experience at all if he hadn't been willing to run a marathon in 5 hours? I don't think so. And to me, that's the point. It's all about the medal.

I've seen people come across the finish line angry and swearing. It's hard to tell exactly whom they're angry with or swearing at, but I'd be willing to guess it is the memory of someone who told them all the things that they would never accomplish.

I've seen people laughing as if they were attending the last show at a comedy club. They're usually so giddy that it's contagious. I find myself laughing right along with them.

Every emotion imaginable comes across the finish line on the shoulders of the participants. And every emotion is valid. Every emotion is worth its weight in gold.

It may sound trite to say that your life can change in a single step. And it would be trite if it wasn't so true. No one who has trained for and started and finished a long-distance event is ever the same person. The changes can be subtle and they aren't all obvious at first, but they're there. Sooner or later the effects are felt.

The Courage to Start

As we've said all along, the most difficult part of any long-distance training program isn't finishing the race. For most of us, getting to the finish line is almost a forgone conclusion. After all, if we've trained well and don't have any major mishaps, there's almost no reason not to finish.

The most difficult part of the training program is getting to the starting line. You must confront so many obstacles. There are so many places for things to go wrong, so many times when you can give up and quit, that, if you are there when the gun goes off, you are already a different person than when you took your first training run.

Right now, as you read this, millions of other people also want to walk or run a half-marathon or marathon. They dream about it at work, in the car, or while watching television. They know just how they want it to be. They think they know what the training will be like, what their bodies will look like, what the race will be like, and how it will feel to stand at the starting line. They even believe that they know how it will feel to cross the finish line.

But they're just dreaming. They aren't doing it. You are. On race morning, when you are out there standing at the starting line with your number on, surrounded by others just like you, you will know what they only imagine. You will feel it, see it, smell it, and experience it. Unlike those who only dream, you've earned the right to be a part of the experience.

By getting to the starting line, you've already placed yourself in the top echelon of athletes. You may not be in the top tier of that race, but as a long-distance athlete, you are fitter, better trained, and more disciplined than 99 percent of the population that has ever lived. Remind yourself of that when you start to obsess about your pace or finish time.

When you stand at the starting line, you join the club. When you stand at the starting line, you earn your membership. Millions dream of being where you are. You are no longer a dreamer. You are a doer.

Thousands more started a training program but never finished. They started with the same enthusiasm (or more than) you had. They started with more or less the same physical gifts or disadvantages that you did. They had no more and no less reason to be successful than you.

But somewhere along the way, they lost that enthusiasm. Somewhere on the road or on the track or treadmill, they decided that the rewards just weren't worth the effort. They decided that they could live without finding their limits, without challenging their expectations of themselves, and without taking a hard look at their image of themselves.

You didn't. If you're standing at the starting line, you've not only accepted the challenge, but you've beaten back the demons. You've conquered your imagination and self-imposed limitations. You've gone farther, gotten stronger, and gotten tougher than you ever imagined.

Though reasons why people don't get to the starting line are many and varied, one particular reason tends to surface over and over. People fail to reach the starting line because they can't, or won't, put their egos aside and listen. They convince themselves that they can do it their way. More often than not, they discover that their ignorance is both dangerous and damaging.

The miracle truly isn't that you are going to finish, but that you had the courage to start—not just the courage to start the race, but the courage to start this odyssey of training and self-discovery. You've had the courage to find out whether you are who you think

Mortal Miracle

"I had always been the kind of person who never finished things. I have dozens of half-read books and magazines. Halfway through training for my first marathon, I wanted to quit. I forced myself to finish. Now running marathons allows me to celebrate my life and my health. Every step, even at mile 24 with fat sausage fingers and sore feet, tells me that I am healthy and strong and will not quit!"

–Belynda, age 31

you are. And if you discovered some new strength, you learned to trust it.

More important, if you discovered some new weakness, you understood that it was just a matter of time and training before that weakness was gone. The medal that you receive for finishing is symbolic of that courage and that willingness. It becomes a powerful icon in your life. Once they place that medal around your neck, no one can ever make you give it back.

Wear It Proudly

What you decide to do with that medal is up to you. We recommend that you wear it until you have annoyed everyone in your life. Wear it to work. Wear it to school. Wear it to bed. Wear it everywhere. Show it to everyone. Tell everyone how you earned it. And don't take it off until someone pries it from your fingers.

The gift of finishing is available to everyone standing at the starting line. It's available if you have the good sense (and good luck) to get out of your own way and achieve what you are capable of achieving. It's available to everyone who is willing to accept who they are at that moment—not who they want to be or wanted to be, but who they are.

Some of you are 3-hour marathoners. Some are 5½-hour marathoners. The differences between you aren't related to your paces. The differences between you are related to genetics, the decisions you've made, and the priorities you have. Your accomplishments, however, are identical.

Everyone who crosses the finish line has earned and deserves a medal. The distance from the starting line to the finish line is the same for everyone. But what we know—and you now know, too—is that the distance from where we are in our life to the

Mortal Miracle

"Running a marathon is like winning an Oscar. Once you've
done it, for the rest of your life, you can say that you are an
Oscar winner. You've had a glimpse of the glory, and you've
earned the title of 'marathoner.' And like the Oscars, you want
to thank everyone who ever helped you reach a goal.

"I ran the Philadelphia marathon in 1999. I dedicated each
mile of the race to someone I loved. The thought of each one
of them got me through that race. The marathon serves as one
of my happiest memories, and even 3 years later, I think of it
when I face a challenge. 'I've run a marathon. . . . I can do this.'"

—Esther, no age given

starting line is different for every one of us. For some, the
starting line may be the next logical step. For others, like us, we
couldn't even see the starting line from where we were in our
lives.

Whatever it took to get to the starting line, leave it all behind
you once the gun goes off. There's no place out on the course for
negative messages, no room in your mind for discouraging
thoughts, no place in your race for old tapes of everything you used
to be or never were. Once you're on the course, you are a long-distance
athlete—nothing more, but nothing less.

You are entitled to the cheers from the crowd. You are entitled
to the pride that you feel when they yell encouragement to you. You
are entitled to believe that you really are looking good, even if
you're sure you aren't. You are entitled to the looks of shock and
disbelief as you keep going mile after mile.

There is no correlation between the time it takes you to finish and the joy that you will experience. There is no formula that predicts how much better you'll feel for every minute (or hour) that you take off your finish time. There is no quid pro quo between speed and satisfaction.

This belief or, some would say, philosophy is often misunderstood. Some critics have chosen to believe that we are encouraging new athletes to do less than their best. Worse critics have even said that we are somehow lowering the bar of excellence in the sport.

We believe that excellence is not a relative term. What is excellent for you has nothing to do with what is excellent for someone else. There may be absolute standards of measurement to determine finishing order. In that setting, it's true that someone crosses the finish line first and someone crosses it last. But that doesn't mean that second place is the first loser.

You are going to discover your personal best somewhere during the training or during the race. There will come a point when you know that you are accomplishing the most that your body, your mind, and your will have to offer. There will come a point when what you believe about yourself equals what is true about yourself.

That can happen at a 5-minute pace or a 15-minute pace. That convergence of belief and reality can happen to anyone at any pace in any race at any distance. Yet it seems as if the longer distances give many of us the time we need to dig deep enough to find the answers that have eluded us.

What you will experience when you cross that first finish line is a physical, emotional, and, some would say, spiritual moment that is unlike any other. That moment is the same whether you finish a full marathon in 3 hours or a half-marathon in 3 hours. Your joy, your satisfaction, your release is not connected to your watch. Your spirit doesn't know how to tell time.

Know Before You Go

Savor that finisher's medal. You earned it! Wear it out the evening after your marathon. Display it for all to see. Smile when people congratulate you on your success. And use it to remind yourself of your accomplishment. If you can do this, you can do anything!
Remember:

- You can't finish if you don't start.
- When in doubt, be conservative.
- The finish line, like the truth, is out there somewhere.
- There will come a moment when you know you will finish.
- Slow down.
- Let yourself feel whatever you feel.
- Don't look at your watch when you finish. Your time doesn't matter.
- Your life will change forever when you cross the finish line.
- Ultimately, it all comes down to a single, final step.
- Everyone gets the same medal.
- Wear your medal until you have annoyed everyone in your life.

CHAPTER SIXTEEN

The Postrace Party

You've done it. You've prepared for and completed your event. You've gone further than you ever thought possible. You've accomplished every goal you had at the start. You are a long-distance athlete. What happens next will define you for the rest of your life.

Mortal Dilemma: *I never thought I could be a
long-distance athlete. Now that I've finished my race,
I feel lost and let down. For months I had a goal that required
my life to be structured. Now that I've accomplished my goal,
what do I do?*

One of the most frequently asked questions is the simplest: Now what? When you've done the impossible, when you've exceeded your wildest expectations, when you've found yourself on the other side of your dream, it's easy to feel lost. If it's any consolation, understand that what you're feeling is normal and healthy.

For months your life has been neatly divided into what you should do to stay on your training program and what you shouldn't do. Now, the morning after the race, that organizing scheme is gone.

All of us who have trained for a major event have felt this way, this empty. The noise and thrill of finishing doesn't last very long. You can spend 6 months preparing but only 3, 6, or more hours racing.

—m—

This may help explain why these days I, John, try to stay out on the course as long as I possibly can. I'm not kidding. I usually start to get depressed at the halfway point of a big event. I know that I've already had half the fun I'm going to have that day.

If this was your first major athletic accomplishment, the feeling of emptiness and loss will seem especially strong. For me, finishing my first marathon began a confusing and frustrating process of having to rethink all of my beliefs about myself. As I began to tell people about having completed a marathon, it became more and more difficult not to think of myself as a long-distance athlete. And if I had become a long-distance athlete, then I'd have to drop all the old images I had of myself.

It's not easy to let go of those old images. I heard a woman once describe herself to me as a "marathoner," not a "runner." "What's the difference?" I asked. She went on to tell me that even though she had completed 12 marathons, she was still heavier than she wanted to be, slower than she wanted to be, and waiting for the magic day when she would be transformed into a runner.

It was a sad moment. Her negative image of herself was so strong that she couldn't let it go even after completing 12 marathons. Her denial about who she had become was so obvious that it was hard to believe that she didn't see it. She didn't. In her mind, staying who she'd always been was more important than accepting who she had become.

Welcome to the Club!

Once you cross that finish line, you join the club. You've earned your membership in the Association of Long-Distance Athletes. Whether you finished first, last, or somewhere in the middle, you belong. Everything that happens next has to start from there. You've done it. In between the starting line and the finish line, you became a different person.

What will that new you do next? It doesn't matter what the old you would have done. That old you is long gone. That old you is lying on the street along with hundreds of empty water cups. That old you disappeared during the thousands of steps you took in training and in the race. The old you no longer exists.

Mortal Miracle

"I feel as though I am walking sideways on the ceiling when I complete a marathon. It's this awesome comforting feeling. Running has made me look at life in a totally different kind of way. I am more tolerable of people and actually catch myself smiling a lot! I feel good about myself inside and out and really enjoy the feeling of freedom when I go for a run.

"I do three marathons a year and will hopefully keep it up until I get old. (When that will be, who knows!)"

—Penelope, age 50

—ɰ—

It's hard to let go of those old images of ourselves. After all, we've carried them around with us for years. Before I, John, finished my first marathon, I always believed that I was not athletic. Thirty-three marathons later I still have to convince myself that I am an athlete. If I'm not careful, all those old messages creep into my thoughts and I'll let myself believe that what used to be true is still true.

Now that you've finished your race and achieved your goal, you need to continue your journey. Step one: Let your body recover. There are lots of ways to do that, and you may have to experiment some before you know what works best for you.

I treat a long-distance race like an auto accident. I'm not kidding. I know that my body has taken a beating, I know that I've done damage to my body, and I know that it's going to take time to heal. I also know now that what hurts a day or two after the event is only the obvious. It can take days or weeks to find out everything that's been affected by the distance.

In the first few days I just try to relax and listen to my body and my soul. If I'm listening carefully, my body will tell me what it needs. And if I listen really carefully, I can hear my soul whispering, too.

Right After You Cross the Line

Coach Jenny will now take you step by step through the rehydration, refueling, and recovery process.

As soon as you can, replace what your body has lost. In the hours and days immediately following a major event, you need to rehydrate, replace electrolytes, repair torn muscles, and restore some kind of balance to your systems. The process begins the instant you cross the finish line.

No matter how well you think you stayed hydrated during the race, you probably still need to replace fluids. It doesn't matter if it was a hot or cold day; you've lost essential body fluid.

It's tempting to just grab the first thing that comes to mind. For some, that would be an ice cold beer or, for John, a hot cup of coffee. But your body really needs water and an electrolyte replacement drink. There's no need to overdo it, but you should start sipping on water and a sports drink as soon as you can.

Eating something salty, like pretzels or potato chips, will help you to get some sodium back into your system. If you can handle crunching away at real food like that, then just do it. In that first 30 minutes it doesn't really matter how you start replacing the electrolytes such as sodium and potassium; it only matters that you do it.

An hour or so after you've finished, start eating protein so that your body can go to work repairing your damaged muscles. And don't think that you have to be sore and tired to have done damage. Even if you feel great at first, get protein into your system.

If you can tolerate them, foods like low-fat yogurt or cottage cheese provide good sources of protein. They'll also help by providing a little calcium, too. Again, it's not a matter of eating lots of anything, but more a matter of eating some of something.

Later, you may find it easier to think about higher protein sources like meat, chicken, or fish. Eat these foods in as pure a form as possible. Avoid consuming anything that's covered in a rich sauce, for example.

Physically, avoid anything that will make your body swell up. We know that a hot shower is sooo inviting, but it's one of the worst things you can do. And sitting for an hour in a hot tub will only bring on a severe case of rigor mortis.

The science behind avoiding the heat is not very exciting.

Simply put, your body—all the joints, muscles, tendons, etc.—are flooded with blood after a rigorous activity like a half- or full marathon. Every part of you is stretched to the limit.

Heat will only cause those already swollen parts to swell even more. And there's nothing worse than waking up the morning after a long race feeling like the Pillsbury Doughboy.

Standing in a lukewarm shower is fine, but sitting in a tub of cool water is even better. It sounds awful, I'm sure. It may not even feel all that good as you lower yourself into the tub. But take our word for it: You'll be glad you did it.

1 Week Postrace

For optimal body recovery, follow the reverse taper outlined in your training program. The first week after your goal event doesn't count. What you do or don't do that week is mostly the result of what happened on race day. And it will be different after different events. If you had one of those golden days, you may feel like getting out and running or walking in as little as 1 week. If you traveled through a gut-wrenching nightmare, you may want to spend the week watching television.

No matter what, during the first few weeks, stick with the post-race recovery workouts listed in your schedule, listen to your body, and let pain be your guide. Add mileage and time gradually. Whatever time you spent running or walking the week before the event is what you should aim for 1 week after the event.

Keep your intensity easy. It will make you feel good to get out and move, but pushing yourself too hard too soon will be hard on your body and your soul.

A word of caution: Don't trust your emotions during this week. So many times a new long-distance athlete finishes and says,

"That's it! I'll never do that again!" Those of us with more experience know that it takes just a few days of recovery before that "never again" mind-set wears way.

2 Weeks and Counting

One to two weeks or so after the event, I'll usually try to go for what amounts to a normal run or walk. In my case, I'll shorten the run interval and do something like a run 3 minutes/walk 1 minute sequence just to see how my legs feel. I'll try to go out for at least 30 minutes but no longer than an hour.

I am always surprised by how hard it feels. I find myself wondering how in the world I could have run a marathon (or half-marathon) just a week before when now I can barely run for 3

Mortal Miracle

"I live on a farm with sheep, pigs, Angora goats, Angora rabbits, cats, dogs, chickens, and some horses. I am the mother of four and have a beautiful 3-year-old granddaughter. Three years ago I finally decided to quit smoking. When I quit smoking I decided to mark my success by running a marathon.

"It was great. It took me more than 5 hours but left me with a feeling I can't describe. My sister really felt my excitement and decided that she was going to quit smoking and run a marathon with me the following year. That marathon took us more than 5 hours and once again I finished with such exhilaration. We were on top of the world."

—Donna, age 43

minutes without getting winded. It's the strangest sensation. I know what I've done. I know I'll do it again, but that first attempt at working out after a big event is always hard on the ego.

An old rule of thumb holds that our bodies need 1 day of recovery for every mile raced. So, for a half-marathon we'd need about 2 weeks, and for a marathon we'd need about a month. It's not that we couldn't run or walk for that long, but that we shouldn't do any long or intense workouts for that length of time.

As the running community has aged, that rule has changed. If you're over 40, you'll probably need a day for every kilometer that you've raced. If you've participated in a half-marathon (21 kilometers) you'll need 3 weeks of recovery, and if you've participated in a marathon (42 kilometers) you'll need up to 6 weeks of recovery—yes, 6 weeks!

The worst mistake you can make—both physically and mentally— is not giving yourself time to recover.

The Postmarathon Blues

For many of us, the physical recovery is easier than the emotional recovery. For some reason, the Wednesday after a big Sunday event is always the worst. I hate the Wednesday syndrome. And no matter how often I race or how many times I experience it, it never feels good.

On race day, the euphoria carries you along like rushing white water. You've got your medal, you're glowing from the accomplishments, and your friends and family are treating you like you've just won a world championship. On Monday morning there's some letdown, but you wear the soreness in your body like a badge of courage. Even if you are banged up, even if you are struggling to get up and down the stairs, you know that it was all for a good reason. The fatigue serves as a reminder of what you achieved.

On Tuesday, it starts to get a little cloudy. Often you are back into your prerace routine of work and family. The spouse and kids begin to tell you all the things you missed while you were training, and the boss wants to know if you've got this long-distance bug out of your system because there's a big project coming up and you'll need to be putting in extra time at work.

All those little tasks and "to-dos" that you postponed during your training are suddenly coming due.

By Wednesday, for us at least, we find ourselves longing to be back out on the racecourse. On the racecourse, we knew who we were. On the racecourse, we were athletes first and everything else second. On the racecourse, we were alone but in the company of friends. On the racecourse, life was simple; just take it one step at a time.

And that's the grand lesson to be learned from preparing for, and participating in, a long-distance event. You've learned that your life as an athlete came down to taking each mile one step at a time. You have the chance to learn that life can be lived in exactly the same way: one step at a time.

You may find that if you're open to it, your training and your race can become a metaphor for living. You've learned that control is an illusion. You can't be more than you are, but you also can't accept less than your potential. You've come to understand that real growth develops not from the stress of activity but from the calmness of recovery.

You come to see that living is a long-distance event. Every day is a training day in one way or another. You may not have understood that when you began the program, but you do now. You've learned how to assess your strengths and weaknesses with honesty and courage. You've learned to acknowledge those strengths and weaknesses without pride or embarrassment.

You've learned that you must acquiesce to the truth about your body and your mind but that you needn't concede to it. You can see who you are today and still hold on to the vision of who you want to be tomorrow.

You've learned that your past is only a description of where you've been, not a prescription for where you will be. You've learned that the choices you've made up to now were based on the best information you had, but that the information was flawed at best or erroneous at worst.

You've learned how to create yourself, to reinvent yourself, to congratulate yourself, and to celebrate yourself. Those lessons don't have to stop just because you've completed your training.

The Rest of Your Life

The finish line is not the end. The finish line is the beginning. Standing at the starting line gives you permission to hope. Taking the time to train, putting in the mileage, making the changes in your life, and taking the risks has given you consent to hope for the best in yourself. The miracle is not that you finished, but that you had the courage to start.

Crossing the starting line also gives you permission to dream. You can dream about the perfect day, the perfect race, and the perfect experience. It may not happen that way, but it doesn't mean you shouldn't dream about it.

Crossing the starting line may be an act of courage, but crossing the finish line is an act of faith. And faith is one of the most powerful emotions you can experience.

Faith is what keeps us going when nothing else will. Faith is the emotion that conquers fear. Faith is the emotion that will give you victory over your past, the demons in your soul, and all of those voices that tell you what you can and cannot do and can and cannot be.

If standing at the starting line gives you permission to dream, crossing the finish line gives you permission to plan. Crossing the finish line gives you permission to plan for your next success, to plan for the realization of your next dream. The last step of the race is the first step of the rest of your life.

What you do now is up to you. You've seen what you can do. If you've stuck with the training program, you've seen yourself filled with joy and blinded by frustration. You've overcome your fears. You've been humbled by both the strength and fragility of your body. You've found what you thought were your limits and gone beyond them.

You've also learned that what stops most of us from achieving our dreams—as athletes and as people—are the confines of our imaginations. We can never be more than we imagine we can be. And as long as we restrict ourselves by our imaginations, we forever bind ourselves to our past and blind ourselves to our futures.

Your limits lie behind you now. With that one final step across the finish line, you liberated yourself from everything you ever thought you knew about yourself. You have taken the very first step on the course to your destiny.

Waddle on. . . .

Know Before You Go

You've done it. You've become a long-distance athlete! Say goodbye to that old you and hello to your inner athlete. Say hello to the part of yourself that will take over and continue this fitness journey. Take a moment to think about your next step. What lies in your future as a long-distance athlete?

Whatever path you take, remember:

- Feeling down after a big race is normal.
- Give yourself time to recover.
- The physical recovery is easier than the emotional recovery.
- It takes 3 weeks to recover from a half-marathon, 6 weeks from a full marathon.
- Stay active, but don't train until you feel ready.
- Take the time to savor the accomplishment.
- Let go of all of your old images of yourself.
- The finish line is not the end.
- Crossing the starting line gives you permission to dream.
- Crossing the finish line gives you permission to plan.

Training
Plans

Walk Half-Marathon

Warmup: Walking 5 minutes at an easy pace prior to every workout.

*Form Drills/Strides: After the walking cooldown, perform 4 stride drills by gradually increasing your walking pace for 30 seconds until fast but controlled pace is reached, focusing on form and quick footstrike. Follow with 1 minute of easy walking. Repeat 4 times.

Heart Rate: Using a heart rate monitor, maintain a range between the prescribed percentages, e.g., 65–75% of maximum heart rate.

Day	Monday	Tuesday	Wednesday
Mode	Walk	Cross-Training	Rest
Intensity	Moderate	Moderate	
Heart Rate	60–75%	60–70%	
I-Rate	6–7.5	6–7	
Week 1	30 min	30 min	Rest
Week 2	30 min	30 min	Rest
Week 3	30 min	30 min	Rest
Week 4	40 min	30 min	Rest
Week 5	40 min	40 min	Rest
Week 6	40 min	40 min	Rest
Week 7	50 min	40 min	Rest
Week 8	50 min	40 min	Rest
Week 9	60 min	40 min	Rest
Week 10	60 min	40 min	Rest
Week 11	60 min	40 min	Rest
Week 12	50 min	30 min	Rest
Week 13	40 min	30 min	Rest
Week 14	30 min	30 min	Rest
Postrace Recovery, Week 1	Rest	20 min	Rest
Postrace Recovery, Week 2	40 min	30 min	Rest
Postrace Recovery, Week 3	50 min	40 min	Rest

I-Rate: Rate the level of intensity by how you feel on a scale of 1–10, 1 being at rest and 10 being an all-out level. Use this system to stay in the smart training range listed in the training program, e.g., 6–7.

Cooldown: Walking 5 minutes at an easy pace after every workout.

Stretch: After every workout when the muscles are warm to maintain or improve flexibility and prevent injuries.

Thursday	Friday	Saturday	Sunday
Walk-Form Moderate 60–75% 6–7.5	Cross-Training Moderate 60–70% 6–7	Endurance Walk Conversational Pace 60–75% 6–7.5	Rest
30 min*	30 min	2 miles	Rest
30 min*	30 min	3 miles	Rest
30 min*	30 min	4 miles	Rest
30 min*	30 min	5 miles	Rest
40 min*	30 min	3 miles	Rest
40 min*	30 min	6 miles	Rest
40 min*	30 min	7 miles	Rest
50 min*	30 min	4 miles	Rest
50 min*	30 min	8 miles	Rest
50 min*	30 min	6 miles	Rest
50 min*	30 min	10 miles	Rest
40 min*	30 min	8 miles	Rest
40 min*	30 min	5 miles	Rest
30 min*	Rest	20 min	Half-marathon
30 min	Rest	2 miles	Rest
40 min	30 min	3 miles	Rest
50 min	30 min	4 miles	Rest

Walk/Run Half-Marathon

Warmup: Walking 5 minutes at an easy pace prior to every workout.

Walk/Run: Walk briskly for prescribed number of minutes and follow with running at a comfortable pace for prescribed number of minutes. Example: "Walk 3 min/Run 1 min Repeat 5 times" means walk briskly for 3 minutes followed by running for 1 minute; repeat sequence 5 times for a total of 20 minutes plus warmup and cooldown.

*Form Drills/Strides: After the walking cooldown, perform 4 stride drills by gradually increasing your walking pace for 30 seconds until fast but controlled pace is reached, focusing on form and quick footstrike. Follow with 1 minute of easy walking. Repeat 4 times.

Day	Monday	Tuesday	Wednesday
Mode	Walk/Run	Cross-Training	Rest
Intensity	Moderate	Moderate	
Heart Rate	60–75%	60–70%	
I-Rate	6–7.5	6–7	
Week 1	32 min: Walk 3 min/ Run 1 min Repeat 8 times	30 min	Rest
Week 2	32 min: Walk 3 min/ Run 1 min Repeat 8 times	30 min	Rest
Week 3	32 min: Walk 3 min/ Run 1 min Repeat 8 times	30 min	Rest
Week 4	32 min: Walk 3 min/ Run 1 min Repeat 8 times	30 min	Rest
Week 5	40 min: Walk 3 min/ Run 1 min Repeat 10 times	30 min	Rest
Week 6	40 min: Walk 3 min/ Run 1 min Repeat 10 times	40 min	Rest

Heart Rate: Using a heart rate monitor, maintain a range between the pre-scribed percentages, e.g., 65–75% of your estimated maximum heart rate.

I-Rate: Rate of perceived exertion. Rate the level of intensity by how you feel on a scale of 1–10, 1 being at rest and 10 being an all-out level. Use this system to stay in the smart training range listed in the training program, e.g., 6–7.

Cooldown: Walking 5 minutes at an easy pace after every workout.

Stretch: After every workout when the muscles are warm to maintain or im-prove flexibility and prevent injuries.

Thursday	Friday	Saturday	Sunday
Walk/Run-Form Moderate 60–75% 6–7.5	Cross-Training Moderate 60–70% 6–7	Endurance Walk/Run Comfortably Brisk 60–75% 6–7.5	Rest
32 min*: Walk 3 min/ Run 1 min Repeat 8 times	30 min	2 miles: Walk 4 min/ Run 1 min Repeat continuously	Rest
32 min*: Walk 3 min/ Run 1 min Repeat 8 times	30 min	3 miles: Walk 4 min/ Run 1 min Repeat continuously	Rest
32 min*: Walk 3 min/ Run 1 min Repeat 8 times	30 min	4 miles: Walk 4 min/ Run 1 min Repeat continuously	Rest
40 min*: Walk 3 min/ Run 1 min Repeat 10 times	30 min	5 miles: Walk 4 min/ Run 1 min Repeat continuously	Rest
40 min*: Walk 3 min/ Run 1 min Repeat 10 times	30 min	3 miles: Walk 3 min/ Run 1 min Repeat continuously	Rest
40 min*: Walk 3 min/ Run 2 min Repeat 8 times	30 min	6 miles: Walk 3 min/ Run 1 min Repeat continuously	Rest

Walk/Run Half-Marathon (cont.)

Day	Monday	Tuesday	Wednesday
Week 7	48 min: Walk 3 min/ Run 1 min Repeat 12 times	40 min	Rest
Week 8	48 min: Walk 3 min/ Run 1 min Repeat 12 times	40 min	Rest
Week 9	45 min: Walk 3 min/ Run 2 min Repeat 9 times	40 min	Rest
Week 10	50 min: Run 3 min Walk 2 min/ Repeat 10 times	40 min	Rest
Week 11	50 min: Walk 3 min/ Run 2 min Repeat 10 times	40 min	Rest
Week 12	50 min: Walk 3 min/ Run 2 min Repeat 10 times	40 min	Rest
Week 13	40 min: Walk 3 min/ Run 2 min Repeat 8 times	30 min	Rest
Week 14	30 min: Walk 3 min/ Run 2 min Repeat 6 times	30 min	Rest
Postrace Recovery, Week 1	Rest	20 min	Rest
Postrace Recovery, Week 2	40 min W/R 3/2	30 min	Rest
Postrace Recovery, Week 3	50 min: W/R 3/2	40 min	Rest

Thursday	Friday	Saturday	Sunday
40 min*: Walk 3 min/ Run 2 min Repeat 8 times	30 min	7 miles: Walk 3 min/ Run 1 min Repeat continuously	Rest
45 min*: Walk 3 min/ Run 2 min Repeat 9 times	30 min	4 miles: Walk 3 min/ Run 2 min Repeat continuously	Rest
45 min*: Walk 3 min/ Run 2 min Repeat 9 times	30 min	8 miles: Walk 3 min/ Run 1 min Repeat continuously	Rest
50 min*: Walk 3 min/ Run 2 min Repeat 10 times	30 min	6 miles: Walk 3 min/ Run 2 min Repeat continuously	Rest
50 min*: Walk 3 min/ Run 2 min Repeat 10 times	30 min	10 miles: Walk 3 min/ Run 1 min Repeat continuously	Rest
45 min*: Walk 3 min/ Run 2 min Repeat 9 times	30 min	8 miles: Walk 3 min/ Run 2 min Repeat continuously	Rest
40 min*: Walk 3 min/ Run 2 min Repeat 8 times	30 min	5 miles: Walk 3 min/ Run 2 min Repeat continuously	Rest
30 min*: Walk 3 min/ Run 2 min Repeat 6 times	Rest	20 min: Walk 3 min/ Run 1 min Repeat 5 times	Half-marathon Walk: 3 min/ Run: 2 min Repeat continuously
32 min: W/R 3/1	Rest	2 miles: W/R 3/1	Rest
40 min: W/R 3/2	30 min	3 miles: W/R 3/2	Rest
50 min: W/R 3/2	30 min	4 miles: W/R 3/2	Rest

Run/Walk Half-Marathon

Warmup: Walking 5 minutes at an easy pace prior to every workout.

Run/Walk: Run at a conversational pace for prescribed number of minutes and follow with walking at a brisk pace for prescribed number of minutes. Example: "Run 3 min/Walk 2 min Repeat 5 times" means run at a conversational pace for 3 minutes followed by walking briskly for 2 minutes; repeat sequence 5 times for a total of 25 minutes plus warmup and cooldown.

*Form Drills/Strides: After the walking cooldown, perform 4 stride drills by gradually increasing your running pace for 30 seconds until fast but controlled pace is reached, focusing on form and quick footstrike. Follow with 1 minute of easy walking. Repeat 4 times.

Day	Monday	Tuesday	Wednesday
Mode	Run/Walk	Cross-Training	Rest
Intensity	Moderate	Moderate	
Heart Rate	60–75%	60–70%	
i-Rate	6–7.5	6–7	
Week 1	35 min: Run 3 min/ Walk 2 min Repeat 7 times	30 min	Rest
Week 2	35 min: Run 3 min/ Walk 2 min Repeat 7 times	30 min	Rest
Week 3	40 min: Run 3 min/ Walk 2 min Repeat 8 times	30 min	Rest
Week 4	40 min: Run 3 min/ Walk 2 min Repeat 8 times	30 min	Rest
Week 5	45 min: Run 3 min/ Walk 2 min Repeat 9 times	30 min	Rest
Week 6	45 min: Run 3 min/ Walk 2 min Repeat 9 times	30 min	Rest

Heart Rate: Using a heart rate monitor, maintain a range between the pre-scribed percentages, e.g., 65–75% of your estimated maximum heart rate.

I-Rate: Rate of perceived exertion. Rate the level of intensity by how you feel on a scale of 1–10, 1 being at rest and 10 being an all-out level. Use this system to stay in the smart training range listed in the training program, e.g., 6–7.

Cooldown: Walking 5 minutes at an easy pace after every workout.

Stretch: After every workout when the muscles are warm to maintain or im-prove flexibility and prevent injuries.

Thursday	Friday	Saturday	Sunday
Run/Walk-Form Moderate 65–75% 6.5–7.5	Cross-Training Moderate 60–70% 6–7	Endurance Run/Walk Comfortably Brisk 60–75% 6–7.5	Rest
35 min*: Run 3 min/ Walk 2 min Repeat 7 times	30 min	3 miles: Run 3 min/ Walk 2 min Repeat continuously	Rest
35 min*: Run 3 min/ Walk 2 min Repeat 7 times	30 min	4 miles: Run 3 min/ Walk 2 min Repeat continuously	Rest
40 min*: Run 3 min/ Walk 2 min Repeat 8 times	30 min	4 miles: Run 3 min/ Walk 2 min Repeat continuously	Rest
40 min*: Run 3 min/ Walk 2 min Repeat 8 times	30 min	5 miles: Run 3 min/ Walk 2 min Repeat continuously	Rest
45 min*: Run 3 min/ Walk 2 min Repeat 9 times	30 min	5 miles: Run 3 min/ Walk 2 min Repeat continuously	Rest
45 min*: Run 3 min/ Walk 2 min Repeat 9 times	30 min	6 miles: Run 3 min/ Walk 2 min Repeat continuously	Rest

Run/Walk Half-Marathon (cont.)

Day	Monday	Tuesday	Wednesday
Week 7	44 min: Run 3 min/ Walk 1 min Repeat 11 times	30 min	Rest
Week 8	44 min: Run 3 min/ Walk 1 min Repeat 11 times	40 min	Rest
Week 9	44 min: Run 3 min/ Walk 1 min Repeat 11 times	40 min	Rest
Week 10	45 min: Run 4 min/ Walk 1 min Repeat 9 times	40 min	Rest
Week 11	45 min: Run 4 min/ Walk 1 min Repeat 9 times	40 min	Rest
Week 12	45 min: Run 4 min/ Walk 1 min Repeat 9 times	40 min	Rest
Week 13	50 min: Run 4 min/ Walk 1 min Repeat 10 times	30 min	Rest
Week 14	40 min: Run 4 min/ Walk 1 min Repeat 8 times	30 min	Rest
Postrace Recovery, Week 1	Rest	20 min	Rest
Postrace Recovery, Week 2	40 min: R/W 3/1	30 min	Rest
Postrace Recovery, Week 3	40 min: R/W 4/1	40 min	Rest

Thursday	Friday	Saturday	Sunday
44 min*: Run 3 min/ Walk 1 min Repeat 11 times	30 min	7 miles: Run 3 min/ Walk 2 min Repeat continuously	Rest
44 min*: Run 3 min/ Walk 1 min Repeat 11 times	30 min	4 miles: Run 3 min/ Walk 1 min Repeat continuously	Rest
48 min*: Run 3 min/ Walk 1 min Repeat 12 times	30 min	8 miles: Run 3 min/ Walk 2 min Repeat continuously	Rest
45 min*: Run 4 min/ Walk 1 min Repeat 9 times	30 min	6 miles: Run 3 min/ Walk 1 min Repeat continuously	Rest
45 min*: Run 4 min/ Walk 1 min Repeat 9 times	30 min	10 miles: Run 3 min/ Walk 2 min Repeat continuously	Rest
50 min*: Run 4 min/ Walk 1 min Repeat 10 times	30 min	8 miles: Run 3 min/ Walk 1 min Repeat continuously	Rest
45 min*: Run 4 min/ Walk 1 min Repeat 9 times	30 min	5 miles: Run 3 min/ Walk 1 min Repeat continuously	Rest
30 min*: Run 4 min/ Walk 1 min Repeat 6 times	Rest	20 min: Run 3 min/ Walk 1 min Repeat 5 times	Half-marathon Run: 4 min/ Walk: 1 min Repeat continuously
30 min: R/W 3/2	Rest	3 miles: R/W 3/2	Rest
40 min: R/W 3/1	30 min	3 miles: R/W 3/1	Rest
40 min: R/W 4/1	30 min	4 miles: R/W 4/1	Rest

Run Half-Marathon

Warmup: Walking 5 minutes at an easy pace prior to every workout.

*Form Drills/Strides: After the walking cooldown, perform 4 stride drills by gradually increasing your running pace for 30 seconds until fast but controlled pace is reached, focusing on form and quick footstrike. Follow with 1 minute of easy walking. Repeat 4 times.

Heart Rate: Using a heart rate monitor, maintain a range between the prescribed percentages, e.g., 65–75% of maximum heart rate.

Day	Monday	Tuesday	Wednesday
Mode	Run-Easy	Cross-Training	Rest
Intensity	Moderate	Moderate	
Heart Rate	65–75%	60–70%	
I-Rate	6.5–7.5	6–7	
Week 1	30 min	30 min	Rest
Week 2	30 min	30 min	Rest
Week 3	30 min	30 min	Rest
Week 4	30 min	30 min	Rest
Week 5	40 min	40 min	Rest
Week 6	40 min	40 min	Rest
Week 7	50 min	40 min	Rest
Week 8	50 min	40 min	Rest
Week 9	50 min	40 min	Rest
Week 10	60 min	40 min	Rest
Week 11	60 min	40 min	Rest
Week 12	50 min	30 min	Rest
Week 13	40 min	30 min	Rest
Week 14	30 min	30 min	Rest
Postrace Recovery, Week 1	Rest	20 min	Rest
Postrace Recovery, Week 2	30 min	30 min	Rest
Postrace Recovery, Week 3	40 min	40 min	Rest

I-Rate: Rate of perceived exertion. Rate the level of intensity by how you feel on a scale of 1–10, 1 being at rest and 10 being an all-out level. Use this system to stay in the smart training range listed in the training program, e.g., 6–7.

Cooldown: Walking 5 minutes at an easy pace after every workout.

Stretch: After every workout when the muscles are warm to maintain or improve flexibility and prevent injuries.

Thursday	Friday	Saturday	Sunday
Run-Form*	Cross-Training	Endurance Run	Rest
Moderate	Moderate	Conversational Pace	
65–75%	60–70%	60–75%	
6.5–7.5	6–7	6–7.5	
30 min*	30 min	2 miles	Rest
30 min*	30 min	3 miles	Rest
30 min*	30 min	4 miles	Rest
30 min*	30 min	5 miles	Rest
40 min*	30 min	3 miles	Rest
40 min*	30 min	6 miles	Rest
40 min*	30 min	7 miles	Rest
50 min*	30 min	4 miles	Rest
50 min*	30 min	8 miles	Rest
50 min*	30 min	6 miles	Rest
50 min*	30 min	10 miles	Rest
40 min*	30 min	8 miles	Rest
40 min*	30 min	5 miles	Rest
30 min*	Rest	20 min	Half-marathon
30 min	Rest	3 miles	Rest
40 min	Rest	4 miles	Rest
40 min	30 min	5 miles	Rest

Walk Marathon

Warmup: Walking 5 minutes at an easy pace prior to every workout.

*Form Drills/Strides: After the walking cooldown, perform 4 stride drills by gradually increasing your walking pace for 30 seconds until a fast but controlled pace is reached, focusing on form and quick footstrike. Follow with 1 minute of easy walking. Repeat 4 times.

Heart Rate: Using a heart rate monitor, maintain a range between the prescribed percentages, e.g., 60–70% of estimated maximum heart rate.

Day	Monday	Tuesday	Wednesday
Mode	Walk	Cross-Training	Walk/Rest
Intensity	Moderate	Moderate	Moderate
Heart Rate	60–75%	60–70%	60–75%
I-Rate	6–7.5	6–7	6–7.5
Week 1	40 min	30 min	40 min
Week 2	40 min	30 min	40 min
Week 3	40 min	30 min	40 min
Week 4	45 min	30 min	Rest
Week 5	45 min	30 min	45 min
Week 6	45 min	30 min	45 min
Week 7	50 min	40 min	Rest
Week 8	50 min	40 min	45 min
Week 9	50 min	40 min	45 min
Week 10	60 min	40 min	Rest
Week 11	60 min	40 min	45 min
Week 12	60 min	40 min	45 min
Week 13	60 min	40 min	45 min
Week 14	50 min	40 min	Rest
Week 15	60 min	40 min	45 min
Week 16	50 min	40 min	Rest
Week 17	60 min	40 min	45 min
Week 18	50 min	30 min	40 min
Week 19	40 min	30 min	40 min
Week 20	30 min	Rest	30 min
Postrace Recovery, Week 1	Rest	20 min	Rest
Postrace Recovery, Week 2	30 min	30 min	Rest
Postrace Recovery, Week 3	30 min	40 min	30 min

I-Rate: Rate of perceived exertion. Rate the level of intensity by how you feel on a scale of 1–10, 1 being at rest and 10 being an all-out level. Use this system to stay in the smart training range listed in the training program, e.g., 6–7.

Cooldown: Walking 5 minutes at an easy pace after every workout.

Stretch: After every workout when the muscles are warm to maintain or improve flexibility and prevent injuries.

Thursday	Friday	Saturday	Sunday
Walk-Form Moderate 60–75% 6–7.5	Cross-Training Moderate 60–70% 6–7	Endurance Walk Conversational Pace 60–75% 6–7.5	Rest
40 min*	30 min	5 miles	Rest
40 min*	30 min	6 miles	Rest
40 min*	30 min	7 miles	Rest
40 min*	30 min	6 miles	Rest
40 min*	30 min	8 miles	Rest
40 min*	30 min	9 miles	Rest
40 min*	40 min	6 miles	Rest
50 min*	30 min	10 miles	Rest
50 min*	30 min	12 miles	Rest
50 min*	40 min	6 miles	Rest
50 min*	30 min	14 miles	Rest
50 min*	40 min	8 miles	Rest
50 min*	30 min	16 miles	Rest
50 min*	40 min	8 miles	Rest
50 min*	30 min	18 miles	Rest
50 min*	40 min	8 miles	Rest
50 min*	30 min	20 miles	Rest
50 min*	30 min	10 miles	Rest
40 min*	30 min	6 miles	Rest
30 min*	Rest	20 min	Marathon
20 min	20 min	2 miles	Rest
30 min	30 min	3 miles	Rest
30 min	30 min	4 miles	Rest

Walk/Run Marathon

Warmup: Walking 5 minutes at an easy pace prior to every workout.

Walk-Run: Walk briskly for prescribed number of minutes and follow with running at a comfortable pace for prescribed minutes. Example: "Walk 3 min/Run 1 min Repeat 5 times" means walk briskly for 3 minutes followed by running for 1 minute; repeat sequence 5 times for a total of 20 minutes plus warmup and cooldown.

***Form Drills/Strides:** After the walking cooldown, perform 4 stride drills by gradually increasing your walking pace for 30 seconds until a fast but controlled pace is reached, focusing on form and quick footstrike. Follow with 1 minute of easy walking. Repeat 4 times.

Day	Monday	Tuesday	Wednesday
Mode	Walk/Run	Cross-Training	Walk-Form*
Intensity	Moderate	Moderate	Moderate
Heart Rate	60–75%	60–70%	65–75%
I-Rate	6–7.5	6–7	6.5–7.5
Week 1	32 min: Walk 3 min/ Run 1 min Repeat 8 times	30 min	40 min*
Week 2	32 min: Walk 3 min/ Run 1 min Repeat 8 times	30 min	40 min*
Week 3	32 min: Walk 3 min/ Run 1 min Repeat 8 times	30 min	40 min*
Week 4	40 min: Walk 3 min/ Run 1 min Repeat 10 times	30 min	45 min*
Week 5	40 min: Walk 3 min/ Run 1 min Repeat 10 times	30 min	45 min*
Week 6	40 min: Walk 3 min/ Run 1 min Repeat 10 times	30 min	45min*

Heart Rate: Using a heart rate monitor, maintain a range between the pre-scribed percentages, e.g., 65–75% of estimated maximum heart rate.

I-Rate: Rate of perceived exertion. Rate the level of intensity by how you feel on a scale of 1–10, 1 being at rest and 10 being an all-out level. Use this system to stay in the smart training range listed in the training program, e.g., 6–7.

Cooldown: Walking 5 minutes at an easy pace after every workout.

Stretch: After every workout when the muscles are warm to maintain or improve flexibility and prevent injuries.

Thursday	Friday	Saturday	Sunday
Walk/Run	Cross-Training	Endurance Walk/Run	Rest
Moderate	Moderate	Comfortably Brisk	
60–75%	60–70%	60–75%	
6–7.5	6–7	6–7.5	
32 min: Walk 3 min/ Run 1 min Repeat 8 times	30 min	5 miles: Walk 4 min/ Run 1 min Repeat continuously	Rest
32 min: Walk 3 min/ Run 1 min Repeat 8 times	30 min	6 miles: Walk 4 min/ Run 1 min Repeat continuously	Rest
32 min: Walk 3 min/ Run 1 min Repeat 8 times	30 min	7 miles: Walk 4 min/ Run 1 min Repeat continuously	Rest
40 min: Walk 3 min/ Run 1 min Repeat 10 times	30 min	6 miles: Walk 4 min/ Run 1 min Repeat continuously	Rest
40 min: Walk 3 min/ Run 1 min Repeat 10 times	30 min	8 miles: Walk 4 min/ Run 1 min Repeat continuously	Rest
40 min: Walk 3 min/ Run 2 min Repeat 10 times	30 min	9 miles: Walk 4 min/ Run 1 min Repeat continuously	Rest

Walk/Run Marathon (cont.)

Day	Monday	Tuesday	Wednesday
Week 7	48 min: Walk 3 min/ Run 1 min Repeat 12 times	30 min	50 min*
Week 8	48 min: Walk 3 min/ Run 1 min Repeat 12 times	30 min	50 min*
Week 9	48 min: Walk 3 min/ Run 1 min Repeat 12 times	30 min	50 min*
Week 10	45 min: Walk 3 min/ Run 2 min Repeat 9 times	40 min	60 min*
Week 11	45 min: Walk 3 min/ Run 2 min Repeat 9 times	40 min	60 min*
Week 12	50 min: Walk 3 min/ Run 2 min Repeat 10 times	40 min	60 min*
Week 13	50 min: Walk 3 min/ Run 2 min Repeat 10 times	40 min	60 min*
Week 14	48 min: Walk 3 min/ Run 1 min Repeat 12 times	40 min	50 min*
Week 15	50 min: Walk 3 min/ Run 2 min Repeat 10 times	40 min	60 min*
Week 16	48 min: Walk 3 min/ Run 1 min Repeat 12 times	40 min	50 min*

Thursday	Friday	Saturday	Sunday
40 min: Walk 3 min/ Run 2 min Repeat 8 times	30 min	6 miles: Walk 3 min/ Run 1 min Repeat continuously	Rest
40 min: Walk 3 min/ Run 2 min Repeat 8 times	30 min	10 miles: Walk 3 min/ Run 1 min Repeat continuously	Rest
40 min: Walk 3 min/ Run 2 min Repeat 8 times	30 min	12 miles: Walk 3 min/ Run 1 min Repeat continuously	Rest
50 min: Walk 3 min/ Run 2 min Repeat 10 times	30 min	6 miles: Walk 3 min/ Run 1 min Repeat continuously	Rest
50 min: Walk 3 min/ Run 2 min Repeat 10 times	30 min	14 miles: Walk 3 min/ Run 1 min Repeat continuously	Rest
50 min: Walk 3 min/ Run 2 min Repeat 10 times	30 min	8 miles: Walk 3 min/ Run 2 min Repeat continuously	Rest
50 min: Walk 3 min/ Run 2 min Repeat 10 times	30 min	16 miles: Walk 3 min/ Run 1 min Repeat continuously	Rest
50 min: Walk 3 min/ Run 2 min Repeat 10 times	30 min	8 miles: Walk 3 min/ Run 2 min Repeat continuously	Rest
45 min: Walk 3 min/ Run 2 min Repeat 9 times	30 min	18 miles: Walk 3 min/ Run 1 min Repeat continuously	Rest
50 min: Walk 3 min/ Run 2 min Repeat 10 times	30 min	8 miles: Walk 3 min/ Run 2 min Repeat continuously	Rest

Walk/Run Marathon (cont.)

Day	Monday	Tuesday	Wednesday
Week 17	50 min: Walk 3 min/ Run 2 min Repeat 10 times	40 min	60 min*
Week 18	48 min: Walk 3 min/ Run 1 min Repeat 12 times	40 min	50 min*
Week 19	45 min: Walk 3 min/ Run 2 min Repeat 9 times	30 min	40 min*
Week 20	30 min: Walk 3 min/ Run 2 min Repeat 6 times	Rest	30 min*
Postrace Recovery, Week 1	Rest	20 min	20 min
Postrace Recovery, Week 2	32 min: W/R 3/1	30 min	Rest
Postrace Recovery, Week 3	30 min:W/R 3/2	40 min	30 min

Thursday	Friday	Saturday	Sunday
45 min: Walk 3 min/ Run 2 min Repeat 9 times	30 min	20 miles: Walk 3 min/ Run 1 min Repeat continuously	Rest
45 min: Walk 3 min/ Run 2 min Repeat 9 times	30 min	10 miles: Walk 3 min/ Run 2 min Repeat continuously	Rest
45 min: Walk 3 min/ Run 2 min Repeat 9 times	30 min	6 miles: Walk 3 min/ Run 2 min Repeat continuously	Rest
20 min: Walk 3 min/ Run 2 min Repeat 4 times	Rest	16 min Walk 3 min/ Run 1 min Repeat 4 times	Marathon Walk 3 min/ Run 2 min Repeat continuously
Rest	20 min	2 miles: Walk	Rest
32 min: W/R 3/1	30 min	3 miles: W/R 3/1	Rest
30 min: W/R 3/2	30 min	3 miles: W/R 3/2	Rest

Run/Walk Marathon

Warmup: Walking 5 minutes at an easy pace prior to every workout.

Run/Walk: Run at a comfortable pace for prescribed number of minutes and follow with walking at a brisk pace for prescribed number of minutes. Example: "Run 3 min/Walk 2 min Repeat 5 times" means run for 3 minutes followed by walking for 2 minutes; repeat sequence 5 times for a total of 25 minutes plus warmup and cooldown.

*Form Drills/Strides: After the walking cooldown, perform 4 stride drills by gradually increasing your running pace for 30 seconds until a fast but controlled pace is reached, focusing on form and quick footstrike. Follow with 1 minute of easy walking. Repeat 4 times.

Day	Monday	Tuesday	Wednesday
Mode	Run/Walk	Run/Walk	Cross-Training
Intensity	Moderate	Moderate	Moderate
Heart Rate	65–75%	65–75%	60–70%
I-Rate	6.5–7.5	6.5–7.5	6–7
Week 1	35 min: Run 3 min/ Walk 2 min Repeat 7 times	35 min: Run 3 min/ Walk 2 min Repeat 7 times	30 min
Week 2	35 min: Run 3 min/ Walk 2 min Repeat 7 times	35 min: Run 3 min/ Walk 2 min Repeat 7 times	30 min
Week 3	40 min: Run 3 min/ Walk 2 min Repeat 8 times	35 min: Run 3 min/ Walk 2 min Repeat 7 times	30 min
Week 4	40 min: Run 3 min/ Walk 2 min Repeat 8 times	35 min: Run 3 min/ Walk 2 min Repeat 7 times	30 min
Week 5	45 min: Run 3 min/ Walk 2 min Repeat 9 times	40 min: Run 3 min/ Walk 2 min Repeat 8 times	30 min
Week 6	45 min: Run 3 min/ Walk 2 min Repeat 9 times	40 min: Run 3 min/ Walk 2 min Repeat 8 times	30 min

Heart Rate: Using a heart rate monitor, maintain a range between the pre-scribed percentages, e.g., 65–75% of estimated maximum heart rate.

I-Rate: Rate of perceived exertion. Rate the level of intensity by how you feel on a scale of 1–10, 1 being at rest and 10 being an all-out level. Use this system to stay in the smart training range listed in the training program, e.g., 6–7.

Cooldown: Walking 5 minutes at an easy pace after every workout.

Stretch: After every workout when the muscles are warm to maintain or im-prove flexibility and prevent injuries.

Thursday	Friday	Saturday	Sunday
Run/Walk-Form* Moderate 65–75% 6.5–7.5	Rest	Endurance Run/Walk Comfortably Brisk 60–75% 6–7.5	Rest
35 min*: Run 3 min/ Walk 2 min Repeat 7 times	Rest	5 miles: Run 3 min/ Walk 2 min Repeat continuously	Rest
35 min*: Run 3 min/ Walk 2 min Repeat 7 times	Rest	6 miles: Run 3 min/ Walk 2 min Repeat continuously	Rest
40 min*: Run 3 min/ Walk 2 min Repeat 8 times	Rest	7 miles: Run 3 min/ Walk 2 min Repeat continuously	Rest
40 min*: Run 3 min/ Walk 2 min Repeat 8 times	Rest	6 miles: Run 3 min/ Walk 2 min Repeat continuously	Rest
45 min*: Run 3 min/ Walk 2 min Repeat 9 times	Rest	8 miles: Run 3 min/ Walk 2 min Repeat continuously	Rest
45 min*: Run 3 min/ Walk 2 min Repeat 9 times	Rest	9 miles: Run 3 min/ Walk 2 min Repeat continuously	Rest

Run/Walk Marathon (cont.)

Day	Monday	Tuesday	Wednesday
Week 7	44 min: Run 3 min/ Walk 1 min Repeat 11 times	40 min: Run 3 min/ Walk 2 min Repeat 8 times	30 min
Week 8	44 min: Run 3 min/ Walk 1 min Repeat 11 times	40 min: Run 3 min/ Walk 1 min Repeat 10 times	30 min
Week 9	44 min: Run 3 min/ Walk 1 min Repeat 11 times	40 min: Run 3 min/ Walk 1 min Repeat 10 times	30 min
Week 10	45 min: Run 4 min/ Walk 1 min Repeat 9 times	40 min: Run 3 min/ Walk 1 min Repeat 10 times	40 min
Week 11	45 min: Run 4 min/ Walk 1 min Repeat 9 times	40 min: Run 3 min/ Walk 1 min Repeat 10 times	40 min
Week 12	45 min: Run 4 min/ Walk 1 min Repeat 9 times	44 min: Run 3 min/ Walk 1 min Repeat 11 times	40 min
Week 13	50 min: Run 4 min/ Walk 1 min Repeat 10 times	44 min: Run 3 min/ Walk 1 min Repeat 11 times	40 min
Week 14	45 min: Run 5 min/ Walk 1 min Repeat 8 times	40 min: Run 4 min/ Walk 1 min Repeat 8 times	40 min
Week 15	48 min: Run 5 min/ Walk 1 min Repeat 8 times	40 min: Run 4 min/ Walk 1 min Repeat 8 times	40 min

Thursday	Friday	Saturday	Sunday
44 min*: Run 3 min/ Walk 1 min Repeat 11 times	Rest	6 miles: Run 3 min/ Walk 1 min Repeat continuously	Rest
44 min*: Run 3 min/ Walk 1 min Repeat 11 times	Rest	10 miles: Run 3 min/ Walk 2 min Repeat continuously	Rest
48 min*: Run 3 min/ Walk 1 min Repeat 12 times	Rest	12 miles: Run 3 min/ Walk 2 min Repeat continuously	Rest
45 min*: Run 4 min/ Walk 1 min Repeat 9 times	Rest	6 miles: Run 3 min/ Walk 1 min Repeat continuously	Rest
45 min*: Run 4 min/ Walk 1 min Repeat 9 times	Rest	14 miles: Run 3 min/ Walk 2 min Repeat continuously	Rest
50 min*: Run 4 min/ Walk 1 min Repeat 10 times	Rest	8 miles: Run 4 min/ Walk 1 min Repeat continuously	Rest
45 min*: Run 4 min/ Walk 1 min Repeat 9 times	Rest	16 miles: Run 3 min/ Walk 1 min Repeat continuously	Rest
48 min*: Run 5 min/ Walk 1 min Repeat 8 times	Rest	8 miles: Run 4 min/ Walk 1 min Repeat continuously	Rest
48 min*: Run 5 min/ Walk 1 min Repeat 8 times	Rest	18 miles: Run 4 min/ Walk 1 min Repeat continuously	Rest

Run/Walk Marathon (cont.)

Day	Monday	Tuesday	Wednesday
Week 16	48 min: Run 5 min/ Walk 1 min Repeat 8 times	45 min: Run 4 min/ Walk 1 min Repeat 9 times	40 min
Week 17	48 min: Run 5 min/ Walk 1 min Repeat 8 times	45 min: Run 4 min/ Walk 1 min Repeat 9 times	40 min
Week 18	48 min: Run 5 min/ Walk 1 min Repeat 8 times	40 min: Run 4 min/ Walk 1 min Repeat 8 times	40 min
Week 19	48 min: Run 5 min/ Walk 1 min Repeat 8 times	40 min: Run 4 min/ Walk 1 min Repeat 8 times	30 min
Week 20	30 min: Run 4 min/ Walk 1 min Repeat 6 times	30 min: Run 4 min/ Walk 1 min Repeat 6 times	Rest
Postrace Recovery, Week 1	Rest	20 min	20 min
Postrace Recovery, Week 2	30 min: R/W 3/2	30 min	Rest
Postrace Recovery, Week 3	40 min: R/W 3/1	40 min	30 min

Thursday	Friday	Saturday	Sunday
48 min*: Run 5 min/ Walk 1 min Repeat 8 times	Rest	8 miles: Run 5 min/ Walk 1 min Repeat continuously	Rest
48 min*: Run 5 min/ Walk 1 min Repeat 8 times	Rest	20 miles: Run 4 min/ Walk 1 min Repeat continuously	Rest
48 min*: Run 5 min/ Walk 1 min Repeat 8 times	Rest	10 miles: Run 5 min/ Walk 1 min Repeat continuously	Rest
48 min*: Run 5 min/ Walk 1 min Repeat 8 times	Rest	6 miles: Run 5 min/ Walk 1 min Repeat continuously	Rest
30 min*: Run 4 min/ Walk 1 min Repeat 6 times	Rest	20 min: Run 3 min/ Walk 1 min Repeat 5 times	Marathon Run 5 min/ Walk 1 min Repeat continuously
Rest	20 min	2 miles: R/W 3/2	Rest
30 min: R/W 3/2	30 min	3 miles: R/W 3/2	Rest
40 min: R/W 3/1	30 min	4 miles: R/W 3/1	Rest

Run Marathon

Warmup: Walking 5 minutes at an easy pace prior to every workout.

*Form Drills/Strides: After the walking cooldown, perform 4 stride drills by gradually increasing your running pace for 30 seconds until a fast but controlled pace is reached, focusing on form and quick footstrike. Follow with 1 minute of easy walking. Repeat 4 times.

Heart Rate: Using a heart rate monitor, maintain a range between the prescribed percentages, e.g., 65–75% of estimated maximum heart rate.

I-Rate: Rate of perceived exertion. Rate the level of intensity by how you feel on a scale of 1–10, 1 being at rest and 10 being an all-out level. Use this system to stay in the smart training range listed in the training program, e.g., 6–7.

Tempo Speed Workout: Warm up with 5 minutes of brisk walking. Run for 10 minutes at an easy pace. Run at tempo pace for prescribed number of

Day	Monday	Tuesday	Wednesday
Mode	Run-Easy	Cross-Training	Run-Speed/Form*
Intensity	Moderate	Moderate	Moderate-Hard
Heart Rate	65–75%	60–70%	70–80%
I-Rate	6.5–7.5	6–7	7–8
Week 1	40 min	30 min	40 min*
Week 2	40 min	30 min	40 min*
Week 3	40 min	30 min	40 min*
Week 4	45 min	30 min	40 min*
Week 5	45 min	30 min	40 min*
Week 6	45 min	30 min	40 min*
Week 7	50 min	40 min	Tempo C Workout*
Week 8	50 min	40 min	Tempo C Workout*
Week 9	50 min	40 min	40 min*
Week 10	60 min	40 min	Tempo B Workout*
Week 11	60 min	40 min	40 min*
Week 12	60 min	40 min	Tempo B Workout*
Week 13	60 min	40 min	40 min*
Week 14	50 min	40 min	Tempo A Workout*
Week 15	60 min	40 min	40 min*

minutes (A, B, or C workout). Run for 10 minutes at an easy pace. Walk for 5 minutes at an easy pace to cool down.

Tempo Pace: A pace just outside your comfort zone, comfortably hard, in which you can talk in short, choppy sentences. 80% of maximum heart rate and level 8 on I-Rate scale.

Tempo A Workout: Run for 20 minutes continuously at tempo pace.

Tempo B Workout: Run for 10 minutes at tempo pace. Walk for 2 minutes briskly. Run for 10 minutes at tempo pace.

Tempo C Workout: Run for 5 minutes at tempo pace, Walk for 1 minute briskly. Repeat 3 times.

Cooldown: Walking 5 minutes at an easy pace after every workout.

Stretch: After every workout when the muscles are warm to maintain or improve flexibility and prevent injuries.

Thursday	Friday	Saturday	Sunday
Run/Rest Moderate 65–75% 6.5–7.5	Cross-Training Moderate 65–75% 6.5–7.5	Endurance Run Conversational Pace 60–75% 6–7.5	Rest
40 min	30 min	5 miles	Rest
40 min	30 min	6 miles	Rest
40 min	30 min	7 miles	Rest
Rest	30 min	6 miles	Rest
45 min	30 min	8 miles	Rest
45 min	30 min	9 miles	Rest
Rest	40 min	6 miles	Rest
Rest	30 min	10 miles	Rest
45 min	30 min	12 miles	Rest
Rest	40 min	6 miles	Rest
45 min	30 min	14 miles	Rest
Rest	40 min	8 miles	Rest
45 min	30 min	16 miles	Rest
Rest	40 min	8 miles	Rest
45 min	30 min	18 miles	Rest

Run Marathon (cont.)

Day	Monday	Tuesday	Wednesday
Week 16	50 min	40 min	Tempo B Workout*
Week 17	60 min	40 min	40 min*
Week 18	50 min	30 min	Tempo A Workout*
Week 19	40 min	30 min	Tempo B Workout*
Week 20	30 min	Rest	30 min*
Postrace Recovery, Week 1	Rest	30 min	Rest
Postrace Recovery, Week 2	30 min	30 min	Rest
Postrace Recovery, Week 3	40 min	40 min	40 min

Thursday	Friday	Saturday	Sunday
Rest	40 min	8 miles	Rest
45 min	30 min	20 miles	Rest
Rest	30 min	10 miles	Rest
Rest	30 min	6 miles	Rest
30 min	Rest	20 min	Marathon
Rest	30 min	3 miles	Rest
40 min	30 min	4 miles	Rest
40 min	30 min	5 miles	Rest

Index

Boldface page references indicate illustrations.
Underscored references indicate boxed text.